MCQs in Paediatric Surgery

Anindya Niyogi • Ashok Daya Ram

MCQs in Paediatric Surgery

Revision for Postgraduate Exams

Springer

Anindya Niyogi
King's College Hospital
London, UK

Ashok Daya Ram
Norfolk and Norwich University Hospital
Norwich, UK

ISBN 978-3-031-94123-8   ISBN 978-3-031-94124-5 (eBook)
https://doi.org/10.1007/978-3-031-94124-5

© The Editor(s) (if applicable) and The Author(s), under exclusive license to Springer Nature Switzerland AG 2025

This work is subject to copyright. All rights are solely and exclusively licensed by the Publisher, whether the whole or part of the material is concerned, specifically the rights of translation, reprinting, reuse of illustrations, recitation, broadcasting, reproduction on microfilms or in any other physical way, and transmission or information storage and retrieval, electronic adaptation, computer software, or by similar or dissimilar methodology now known or hereafter developed.
The use of general descriptive names, registered names, trademarks, service marks, etc. in this publication does not imply, even in the absence of a specific statement, that such names are exempt from the relevant protective laws and regulations and therefore free for general use.
The publisher, the authors and the editors are safe to assume that the advice and information in this book are believed to be true and accurate at the date of publication. Neither the publisher nor the authors or the editors give a warranty, expressed or implied, with respect to the material contained herein or for any errors or omissions that may have been made. The publisher remains neutral with regard to jurisdictional claims in published maps and institutional affiliations.

This Springer imprint is published by the registered company Springer Nature Switzerland AG
The registered company address is: Gewerbestrasse 11, 6330 Cham, Switzerland

If disposing of this product, please recycle the paper.

Preface

Examinations are an integral part of every trainee's journey toward advancing their career. Across the globe, written assessments—particularly multiple-choice questions (MCQs)—form the cornerstone of the initial phase of postgraduate examinations in paediatric surgery.

There is no substitute for hard work. Success in these examinations demands a rigorous combination of dedicated reading, continuous practice, and active engagement in clinical work. This book is not intended to be an exhaustive or definitive guide to the first part of the examination. Rather, it is designed to provide trainees with a snapshot of the high standards expected and to inspire further, in-depth exploration of all facets of paediatric surgical practice.

The MCQs presented aim to enhance critical thinking, guiding readers to extract relevant information from textbooks and scientific literature, and apply it in a way that reflects higher-order cognitive skills. We hope this resource serves as a valuable stepping stone, aiding trainees as they delve deeper into each topic in preparation for their examinations.

This book is the product of our own shared journey of preparing for postgraduate exams. Our primary motivation is to support the next generation of paediatric surgeons in achieving their examination goals. More importantly, we believe that the knowledge and skills developed during this process will contribute to the making of not only competent but compassionate surgeons. As our mentors often reminded us, the more proficient a surgeon becomes, the more natural it is to practice with kindness and humility.

While it is impossible to acknowledge every mentor who has influenced and supported us, we remain deeply grateful for their guidance and hope that this work reflects their teachings. We also extend heartfelt thanks to our families and loved ones for their unwavering support, particularly during our most challenging moments.

Above all, this book is dedicated to the smallest and mightiest patients—the surgical infants and children we care for each day—and to their families, who allow us the honour of being part of their extraordinary journeys. We also remember with respect and humility those little lives who, despite not surviving, taught us invaluable lessons that no textbook ever could.

We accept full responsibility for the content of this book and acknowledge that paediatric surgery is a continually evolving field. As such, current best practices may shift with new evidence and experience.

We sincerely hope this book proves to be a helpful companion in your exam preparation and that it plays a part in shaping you into a brilliant and compassionate paediatric surgeon—one who serves with skill, empathy, and dedication.

London, UK Anindya Niyogi
Norwich, UK Ashok Daya Ram

Contents

1 **Fetal Medicine** 1
   Anindya Niyogi and Ashok Daya Ram

2 **Paediatric Trauma** 5
   Anindya Niyogi and Ashok Daya Ram

3 **Oncology** 9
   Anindya Niyogi and Ashok Daya Ram
   3.1   Wilms' Tumour 9
   3.2   Neuroblastoma 11
   3.3   Tumours of the Liver 13
   3.4   Paediatric Gastrointestinal Tumours 16
   3.5   Rhabdomyosarcoma 18
   3.6   Extragonadal Germ Cell Tumours 19
   3.7   Ovarian Tumours 21
   3.8   Testicular Tumours 23
   3.9   Adrenal Tumours 25
   3.10 Tumours of the Lung and Chest Wall 27

4 **Head and Neck** 29
   Anindya Niyogi and Ashok Daya Ram
   4.1   Craniofacial Anomalies 29
   4.2   Salivary Glands 30
   4.3   Lymph Node Disorders 31
   4.4   Thyroid and Parathyroid glands 32
   4.5   Neck Cysts and Sinuses 33

5 **Thorax** 35
   Anindya Niyogi and Ashok Daya Ram
   5.1   Disorders of the Breast 35
   5.2   Congenital Chest Wall Deformities 37
   5.3   Congenital Diaphragmatic Hernia and Eventration 39
   5.4   Congenital Lung Malformations 41
   5.5   Oesophageal Rupture and Perforation 43
   5.6   Oesophageal Atresia 45

	5.7	Foreign Body Ingestion	48
	5.8	Gastroesophageal Reflux Disease	50
6	**Abdomen**		53
	Anindya Niyogi and Ashok Daya Ram		
	6.1	Congenital Defects of the Abdominal Wall	53
	6.2	Inguinal Hernias and Hydroceles	54
	6.3	Undescended Testis	56
	6.4	Pyloric Stenosis	57
	6.5	Bariatric Surgery in Adolescents	59
	6.6	Intestinal Atresia	60
	6.7	Meconium Ileus	62
	6.8	Intussusception	65
	6.9	Malrotation	66
	6.10	Short Bowel Syndrome	68
	6.11	Gastrointestinal Bleeding	69
	6.12	Alimentary Tract Duplications	70
	6.13	Polypoid Diseases of the Gastrointestinal Tract	71
	6.14	Necrotising Enterocolitis	73
	6.15	Inflammatory Bowel Disease	75
	6.16	Appendicitis	78
	6.17	Hirschsprung Disease	79
	6.18	Anorectal Malformations	81
	6.19	Biliary Atresia and Choledochal Cyst	85
	6.20	Gallbladder Disease	88
	6.21	Portal Hypertension	90
	6.22	Pancreas	93
	6.23	Spleen	96
7	**Urology**		101
	Anindya Niyogi and Alok Godse		
	7.1	Renal Agenesis, Dysplasia, and Cystic Disease	101
	7.2	Renal Fusions and Ectopia	104
	7.3	Pelviureteric Junction Obstruction	106
	7.4	Vesicoureteral Reflux	108
	7.5	Urinary Lithiasis	111
	7.6	Renal Infection	113
	7.7	Duplication of Renal Tract	115
	7.8	Disorders of Bladder Function	117
	7.9	Megaureter and Prune-Belly Syndrome	119
	7.10	Bladder and Cloacal Exstrophy	120
	7.11	Hypospadias	121
	7.12	Disorders of Sexual Development	122
	7.13	Posterior Urethral Valves and Urethral Abnormalities	124
Answers			127

Fetal Medicine

1

Anindya Niyogi and Ashok Daya Ram

1. A 34-year-old primigravida mum's second-trimester ultrasound demonstrates that the fetal bowel is brighter than the liver and the surrounding bone.
   What is the most appropriate management?
   A. Parental reassurance with no intervention
   B. Chorionic villus sampling
   C. Follow-up with serial scans
   D. A short trial of maternal steroids
   E. Amniocentesis
2. In a 30-year-old primigravida, a 20-week anomaly scan suggests High Upper Gastrointestinal obstruction in the foetus, and she would like to find out if the baby has any genetic diseases.
   The best investigation would be.
   A. Amniocentesis
   B. Chorionic villus sampling
   C. Foetal MRI
   D. Maternal blood tests.
   E. Parental genetic tests

A. Niyogi (✉)
King's College Hospital, London, UK

A. D. Ram
Norfolk and Norwich University Hospital, Norwich, UK

© The Author(s), under exclusive license to Springer Nature Switzerland AG 2025
A. Niyogi, A. D. Ram, *MCQs in Paediatric Surgery*,
https://doi.org/10.1007/978-3-031-94124-5_1

3. In monochorionic diamniotic twin, the amniotic fluid progressively increases in one and decreases in the other.
   The most appropriate further management is:
   A. Serial imaging till term
   B. Fetoscopic Laser photocoagulation
   C. Amnioinfusion of the smaller sac
   D. Amnioreduction of the larger sac
   E. Termination of the smaller twin
4. 18-year-old mother attended antenatal ultrasound scan at 25 weeks of gestation. The scan demonstrates a left-sided congenital diaphragmatic hernia with no other structural and chromosomal anomaly. In addition, the observed to expected lung-head-ratio is 23%, and there is no liver herniation.
   Which management strategy is most likely to improve survival to discharge from the hospital?
   A. Fetal surgery to repair the diaphragmatic hernia
   B. Perform FETO as soon as possible
   C. Perform FETO at 27–30 weeks of gestation
   D. Serial ultrasound scans with no intervention
   E. Early term delivery at 37 weeks of gestation
5. Ultrasound scan of a foetus at 30 weeks of gestation showed bilateral hydronephrosis, bladder diameter of 30 mm and amniotic fluid index of 10. There are no other abnormalities.
   The most appropriate management plan in this situation is
   A. Vesicoamniotic shunt
   B. Amnioinfusion
   C. Fetal cystoscopy
   D. Maternal steroids
   E. Serial ultrasound
6. A baby was antenatally diagnosed with a Left-sided isolated CPAM with a single dominant cyst. At 28 weeks of gestation, the cyst was enlarging with a CPAM volume ratio (CVR) of 1.8, and the baby developed hydrops.
   What is the most appropriate antenatal management for this baby
   A. Monitor with serial ultrasound
   B. Maternal intravenous betamethasone
   C. Thoracoamniotic shunt
   D. Open fetal surgery
   E. EXIT-to-CPAM resection
7. A baby was prenatally diagnosed with an open lumbar myelomeningocele
   Which treatment strategy is most likely to reduce the need for a ventriculoperitoneal shunt?
   A. Fetal repair before 26 weeks of gestation
   B. Fetal repair after 32 weeks of gestation
   C. Planned premature delivery after 34 weeks of gestation
   D. Postnatal repair
   E. Fetoscopic repair at 30 weeks of gestation

8. A baby with a prenatal diagnosis of predominantly solid sacrococcygeal teratoma developed nonimmune hydrops at 25 weeks of gestation.
   Which of the following has been demonstrated to reduce intrauterine death?
   A. Fetoscopic radiofrequency ablation of feeding vessels
   B. Fetoscopic sclerotherapy of feeding vessels
   C. Fetal debulking surgery
   D. Delivery at 32 weeks
   E. Intrauterine death is inevitable

Paediatric Trauma

2

Anindya Niyogi and Ashok Daya Ram

1. A 6-year-old with blunt abdominal trauma has arrived in the Emergency Department. The pulse rate is 160/min, and the systolic blood pressure is 60 mmHg. The capillary refill is 5 s. An endotracheal tube is already secured, and the chest is rising symmetrically. A large-bore cannula was inserted, and the blood tests were sent.
   The next step in fluid management would be to
   A. Give 450 ml of 0.9% Saline
   B. Give 250 ml of crossed matched blood
   C. Give 400 ml of O negative blood
   D. Give 200 ml of 0.9% Saline
   E. Give 500 ml of Hartmann's solution

2. An 11-year-old boy with blunt abdominal trauma is being resuscitated in the emergency department. Airway and breathing are secured with an endotracheal tube. 2 wide bore cannulas have been inserted, and fluid resuscitation is instituted. The child has received 800 ml of crystalloids and 800 ml of blood in total, and the capillary refill is 5 s with a systolic blood pressure of 60 mmHg.
   The next step in the management is to
   A. Initiate massive transfusion protocol
   B. Trauma laparotomy
   C. Urgent contrast CT scan
   D. FAST scan
   E. Transfer the child to PICU

A. Niyogi (✉)
King's College Hospital, London, UK

A. D. Ram
Norfolk and Norwich University Hospital, Norwich, UK

3. A 4-year-old boy was brought into the emergency department by his parents after a fall from the second floor flat. He is conscious but is very anxious.
   The best initial management of the cervical spine is
   A. Manual in-line stabilisation
   B. Cervical collar
   C. Urgent cervical X-ray
   D. Do nothing
   E. Examination of the spine
4. Another player's knee hit a 12-year-old boy on the left side of the abdomen during a football match yesterday. His CT scan image is shown.

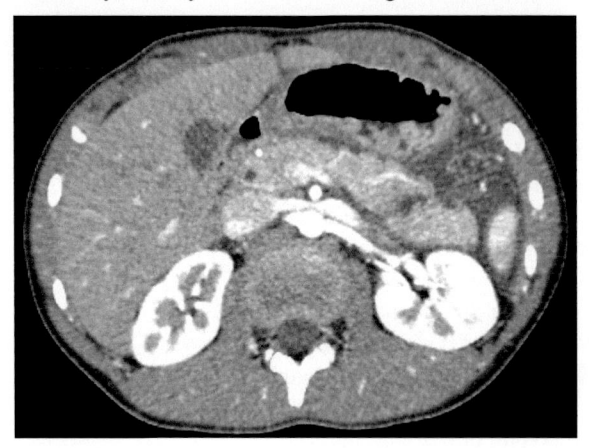

   What is the most appropriate management?
   A. Nasojejunal feeding
   B. Nil by mouth and parenteral nutrition
   C. ERCP and stenting
   D. Distal pancreatectomy
   E. Endovascular embolization
5. After a rugby tackle, an 11-year-old child was admitted to the hospital with a Grade IV splenic laceration. He required 20 ml/kg crystalloids during initial resuscitation to stabilise his vitals. It is the third day following his injury, and his vital signs are normal. He tolerates diet and has minimal abdominal pain. His haemoglobin is 70 g/L today.
   Which is the correct management for this child?
   A. Complete blood count in 6 h
   B. Transfuse packed RBC
   C. Complete five days of bed rest
   D. Repeat imaging before discharge home
   E. Restrict activity for six weeks

6. Blood gas analysis of a 4-year-old child with an isolated head injury shows PaO2 of 8.5 kPa and PaCO2 of 6.5 kPa on air.
   The next step in the management of this child is?
   A. Immediate intubation
   B. 100% Oxygen
   C. 10 ml/Kg normal saline bolus
   D. IV morphine 100 micrograms/kg
   E. Mannitol 0.25–0.5 g/kg
7. A 3-year-old girl sustained a head injury after falling on the wooden floor from the sofa. She lost consciousness for about 10 min after the fall witnessed by her parents. It is now 40 min since the incident, and she is fully alert and playful in the emergency department. No external injuries were identified on examination.
   The next step in the management of the child is?
   A. Observe for a minimum of 4 h
   B. CT scan within 1 h
   C. CT scan within 4 h
   D. Observe for a minimum of 12 h
   E. Discharge home
8. A 1-year-old boy who recently started to walk accidentally pulled a cup of hot coffee on him, resulting in a scald covering the front of the entire chest and abdomen
   The additional fluid (in ml) required per day is
   A. 520
   B. 390
   C. 540
   D. 720
   E. 680
9. A 14-year-old boy sustained a complete posterior urethral disruption associated with a pelvic fracture. Attempt to catheterisation failed
   Which approach will result in the lowest incident of future urethral strictures
   A. Suprapubic drainage and delayed urethroplasty
   B. Primary urethroplasty
   C. Primary endoscopic urethral realignment
   D. Perineal urethrostomy
   E. Suprapubic drainage and delayed endoscopic urethral realignment
10. A hemodynamically stable child with grade IV renal laceration from blunt trauma has ongoing bleeding,
    The recommended treatment is
    A. Conservative
    B. Angioembolisation
    C. Nephrectomy
    D. Ureteric stent
    E. Factor VII infusion

Oncology

3

Anindya Niyogi and Ashok Daya Ram

3.1 Wilms' Tumour

1. A baby born with aniridia and hypospadias is predisposed to early childhood renal tumours.
   Which is the most likely location of genetic mutation in this baby?
   A. 11p15
   B. 11q15
   C. 11p13
   D. 11q13
   E. 13p11
2. During surgery for Wilms tumour, tumour thrombus was resected from the inferior vena cava wall. Histology shows an intermediate-risk stromal subtype.
   What is the UMBRELLA SIOP-RTSG 2016 postoperative treatment?
   A. AV (actinomycin D, doxorubicin) (4 weeks)
   B. AV (actinomycin D, doxorubicin) (27 weeks)
   C. AV (actinomycin D, doxorubicin) (27 weeks) + flank radiotherapy
   D. AVD (actinomycin D, vincristine, doxorubicin) (27 weeks)
   E. AVD (actinomycin D, vincristine, doxorubicin) (27 weeks) + flank radiotherapy
3. A child with WT1 mutation presents with bilateral Wilms Tumour
   Which is the best management plan for this child?
   A. Preoperative chemotherapy to a maximum of 12 weeks followed by bilateral nephron-sparing surgery with less involved kidney operated on first

A. Niyogi (✉)
King's College Hospital, London, UK

A. D. Ram
Norfolk and Norwich University Hospital, Norwich, UK

B. Preoperative chemotherapy to a maximum of 12 weeks followed by nephron-sparing surgery of less involved kidney and radical nephrectomy of the more involved side
C. Preoperative chemotherapy to a maximum of 12 weeks followed by bilateral radical nephrectomy
D. Preoperative chemotherapy for 16 weeks followed by bilateral nephron-sparing surgery with less involved kidney operated on first
E. Preoperative chemotherapy for 16 weeks followed by nephron-sparing surgery of less involved kidney and radical nephrectomy of the more involved side

4. A sampling of lymph nodes during radical nephrectomy for Wilm's tumour is vital for accurate staging and postoperative treatment.
   Which of the following is **not** a correct lymph node sampling strategy?
   A. At least 7 nodes are sampled
   B. Sample inter-aorto-caval nodes for Right-sided tumours
   C. Sample inter-aorto-caval nodes for Left-sided tumours
   D. Sampling of suspicious pre aortic nodes
   E. Radical dissection of all involved nodes

5. A 4-year-old boy has a relapse of Wilms tumour detected 18 months after completing treatment for Wilms tumour.
   Key prognostic factors used to stratify treatment for relapse are
   A. Number and size of metastatic nodules in the lungs.
   B. Histological risk group, tumour stage, and previous treatment intensity
   C. Presence of positive lymph nodes in the abdominal cavity
   D. Age and time of recurrence
   E. Number and size of the recurrence

6. A baby was prenatally diagnosed with a Right renal mass which continued to grow throughout pregnancy. Postnatal MRI suggests a stage III renal tumour. A radical total nephrectomy was performed. Histology showed a cellular subtype of congenital mesoblastic nephroma; however, there was no free margin
   The next step in managing the baby is
   A. No postoperative treatment
   B. Re-resection
   C. 27 weeks of Vincristine and Actinomycin D
   D. 27 weeks of Ifosfamide, Carboplatin and Etoposide
   E. Radiotherapy to the bed

7. A 6-year-old boy with an autosomal dominant familial cancer syndrome associated with a VHL gene mutation in chromosome 3p presents with a stage III renal tumour.
   What is the correct treatment for this particular type of renal cancer?
   A. Pre chemotherapy tumour biopsy
   B. Preoperative high-risk chemotherapy with 5 drugs if a biopsy is unavailable
   C. Same surgical principles as Wilms tumour
   D. AVD chemotherapy postoperatively
   E. No radiotherapy

8. An 11-month-old boy presented with a right renal mass with calcifications and haematuria. He was treated like a Wilms tumour. However, the postoperative histology confirms the most aggressive form of renal malignancy in children. There was no peritoneal contamination.
   Which is the correct management for this child
   A. Neuroimaging
   B. Whole abdomen radiotherapy
   C. Radical lymph node resection
   D. Chemotherapy alone for gross residual tumour
   E. Palliation

3.2 Neuroblastoma

1. An 18-month-old boy presents with neurologic symptoms including spontaneous saccades of the eyes in all directions, involuntary muscle twitching, ataxia and other cerebellar signs. However, he does not have unexplained illness or weight loss.
   The next step in this child's management is:
   A. MRI of the brain
   B. Ophthalmic review
   C. Cross-sectional imaging of chest and abdomen
   D. Referral to a paediatric neurologist
   E. Close observation of symptoms over four weeks.
2. A 2-year-old boy is suspected of having a neuroblastoma relapse after an initial complete treatment of Adrenal neuroblastoma.
   The initial management of the condition is:
   A. Re-biopsy of tumours at the time of relapse at the primary or accessible metastatic site.
   B. Urgent surgical resection of the recurrence.
   C. Immunomodulation therapy.
   D. Myeloablative therapy if received before.
   E. Palliative therapy
3. A 14-month-old girl has isolated CNS relapse following treatment for stage 4 neuroblastoma.
   The next step in the management is:
   A. Palliative care.
   B. Neurosurgical resection of CNS disease.
   C. Chemotherapy with Cyclophosphamide, Vincristine and Doxorubicin.
   D. MIBG therapy
   E. Infusion of anti-GD2 antibody with IL-2

4. A 2-year-old child has suspected left adrenal neuroblastoma in imaging with intraspinal extension and neurologic signs of spinal cord compression with no rapid neurologic deterioration.
   The next step in the management is:
   A. Excision of intraspinal disease
   B. Laminectomy
   C. Removal of the extraspinal tumour
   D. Dexamethasone and Carboplatin/Etoposide
   E. Obtain tissue biopsy before chemotherapy
5. A 2-month-old baby was diagnosed with a localised adrenal masses of 4 cm in diameter, suspicious of neuroblastoma.
   The next step in the management is:
   A. Surgical excision
   B. Ultrasound-guided biopsy
   C. MIBG scan
   D. Bone marrow aspirate
   E. Serial ultrasound and urinary VMA/HVA
6. A 10-month-old baby with stage Ms Neuroblastoma with no segmental chromosomal alterations and no MYCN amplification presented with progressive abdominal distension resulting in breathing difficulties and decreased urine output.
   The management options are all of the following except
   A. Surgical resection
   B. Chemotherapy
   C. Laparostomy
   D. Dexamethasone
   E. Radiotherapy
7. An 18-month-old boy presents with a suspected large left adrenal neuroblastoma displacing the liver and the kidney. The tumour is not encasing any blood vessels, and there is no infiltration into the surrounding structures. However, there is a small ascitis.
   The next step in the management is:
   A. Tumour biopsy
   B. Tumour excision
   C. Carboplatin
   D. Etoposide
   E. Observation
8. A 2-year-old child presents with left adrenal neuroblastoma encasing the aorta and the IVC. Histology shows differentiating cells with no MYCN amplification, and the MIBG scan shows no bony metastasis.
   The next step in the management is:
   A. 4 courses of Carboplatin/Etoposide
   B. 6 courses of CADO (Cyclophosphamide, doxorubicin and vincristine)
   C. Tumour resection
   D. Radiotherapy
   E. 6 courses of 13 cis-retinoic acid

3.3 Tumours of the Liver

1. A baby presents with abdominal mass, thrombocytopenia, and features of hypothyroidism. Her CT is displayed.

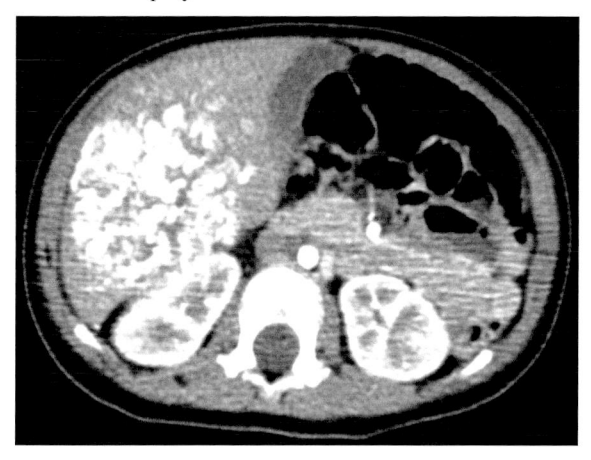

   The options in the management of the baby include all of the following except
   A. Aminocaproic acid
   B. Vincristine
   C. Interferon-alfa
   D. Selective hepatic artery embolization
   E. Radiation therapy

2. An 18-month-old boy presents with abdominal distension. There are no features of high output cardiac failure. The MRI shows a cystic liver lesion as displayed.

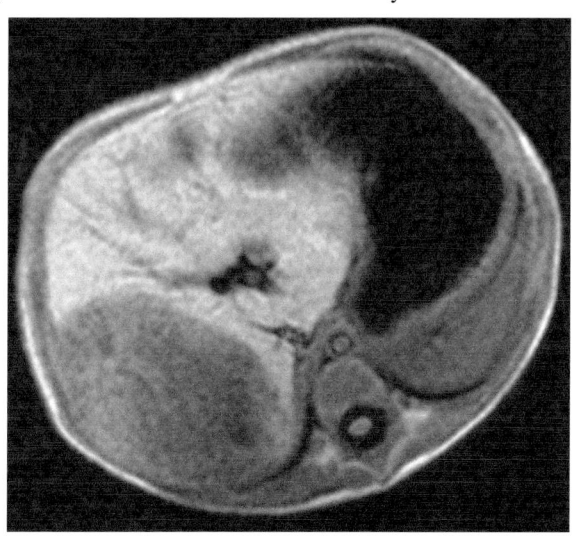

The treatment of choice is
A. Marsupalisation
B. Excision
C. Aspiration
D. Sclerotherapy
E. Liver transplant

3. An adolescent girl, who was successfully treated for neuroblastoma in the past, was found to have a liver mass on surveillance ultrasound. Therefore, a CT scan was performed, which showed an early enhancing lesion with a hypodense central scar as displayed.

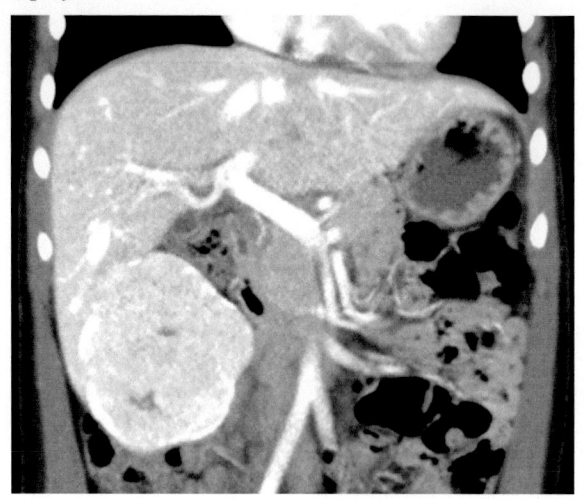

The appropriate management is
A. Serial imaging
B. Resection
C. Arterial embolisation
D. Biopsy
E. Chemotherapy

4. A 2-year-old child diagnosed with a malignant liver tumour has an autosomal dominant genetic condition with a mutation in a gene located in the long arm of chromosome 5 (5q22. 2).
In future, the child is most likely to develop
A. Thyroid cancer
B. Colonic cancer
C. Pancreatic cancer
D. Renal cancer
E. Bone cancer

5. A baby born with hemihypertrophy had transient refractory hypoglycemia after birth.
   Which of the following tumours are least likely to develop?
   A. Wilms Tumour
   B. Hepatoblastoma
   C. Pheochromocytoma
   D. Neuroblastoma
   E. Rhabdomyosarcoma
6. A 4-year-old boy was diagnosed with bilobar, multifocal hepatoblastoma. The AFP level is 75 ng/mL
   What is the next line of management?
   A. Liver transplant
   B. Cisplatin-based chemotherapy
   C. Surgical resection
   D. Chemoembolisation
   E. Radiation therapy
7. A newborn boy presented with hepatic failure and was diagnosed with hereditary tyrosinaemia type I. He was successfully treated with Nitisinone combined with dietary restriction. However, at 18 months of age, his alfa-fetoprotein (AFP) levels started to rise.
   What is the next line of management?
   A. Neoadjuvant chemotherapy
   B. Radiotherapy
   C. Liver transplant
   D. Keep monitoring AFP
   E. Change Nitisinone formulation
8. A 15-year-old girl on contraceptive pills for dysmenorrhoea was incidentally found to have a 4 cm solid liver mass. Alfafetoprotein is normal. The immunohistochemistry of biopsy shows the β-catenin activated HCA (β-HCA) subtype.
   The most appropriate definitive treatment strategy is
   A. Stopping contraceptive pills
   B. Monitor Alfafetoprotein
   C. Serial contrast-enhanced MRI
   D. Radiofrequency ablation
   E. Surgical resection

3.4 Paediatric Gastrointestinal Tumours

1. A 15-year-old boy with Trisomy 21 who had Nissen fundoplication 4 years ago is under surveillance for Barrett's oesophagus. His recent oesophageal biopsy showed oesophageal adenocarcinoma with invasion to the mid submucosa (T1b, sm2)
   Which is the most appropriate treatment?
   A. Endoscopic mucosal resection
   B. Endoscopic radiofrequency ablation
   C. Oesophagectomy
   D. Oesophagectomy, with consideration of neoadjuvant therapy
   E. Oesopagogastrectomy
2. A teenage girl presents with gastrointestinal bleeding, epigastric pain, headaches, fatigue, hypertension and tachycardia. An upper abdominal mass was palpable. MRI showed a 2 cm solid mass in the lesser curvature of the stomach with no metastasis. CT of the chest showed a 1 cm cartilaginous mass in the right upper lobe of the lung and a 2 cm mass in the posterior mediastinum. Her lung function test is normal, but Her urinary metanephrine is high.
   The treatment of the child involves all of the following except
   A. Surgical resection of gastric lesion
   B. Surgical resection of lung lesion
   C. Surgical resection of the posterior mediastinal lesion
   D. Phenoxybenzamine
   E. Propranolol
3. A 15-year-old boy presented with ileocolic intussusception. 10 cm of terminal ileum was resected with the lead point. Histology showed the most common type of intestinal lymphoma in children with complete resection. MRI abdomen showed no residual nodal disease, and the child has no other symptoms.
   The management of this child involves all of the following except
   A. Lumbar puncture
   B. Bone marrow aspirate
   C. Two cycles of chemotherapy
   D. Sperm banking
   E. MRI of the central nervous system
4. A 10-year-old boy with refractory functional constipation and soiling underwent an ACE procedure using the appendix. The histology of the appendix tip showed a 1 cm carcinoid tumour with clear margins.
   The next step of management is?
   A. No further treatment
   B. Complete appendicectomy with the removal of mesoappendix
   C. Right hemicolectomy
   D. Right hemicolectomy with biopsy of the regional lymph nodes
   E. Octreotide

3.4 Paediatric Gastrointestinal Tumours

5. You have performed a proctoscopy on a 9-year-old child with episodes of fresh PR bleeding. You find five discrete polyps. You resect one polyp, more than 1 cm in diameter, showing hamartomatous polyp on histology. There is no family history of intestinal polyps.
   The management of this child includes all of the following except
   A. Colonoscopic surveillance every 1–5 years
   B. Endoscopic polypectomy for polyps >10 mm
   C. Genetic testing for SMAD4 and BMPR1A gene mutation
   D. Colectomy in very high polyp burden
   E. Selective COX-2 inhibitors

6. A 15-year old boy who was previously treated for a cerebellar medulloblastoma presents with abdominal pain, bloody diarrhoea and weight loss. Colonoscopy showed multiple colonic polys, which were adenomatous on histology.
   The management of the child is
   A. Celecoxib
   B. Colonoscopic polypectomy
   C. Panproctocolectomy
   D. Upper GI surveillance
   E. Screening for hepatoblastoma

7. A 15-year-old girl presents with lower GI bleeding. She also had dental anomalies, osteomas, a solitary thyroid nodule, and multiple subcutaneous lipomas. Colonoscopy showed 35 polyps.
   The immediate management of this child would include all accept
   A. Sulindac
   B. Carcinoembryonic antigen (CEA) testing
   C. Alpha-fetoprotein (AFP) testing
   D. Restorative proctocolectomy
   E. Yearly colonoscopy

8. You are counselling an 8-year-old child with a family history of Familial adenomatous polyposis (FAP)
   The management of the child would include all accept
   A. Predictive genetic testing at 12–14 years
   B. Commence colonic surveillance at 12–14 years
   C. Commence upper GI surveillance at 12–14 years
   D. No routine screening for hepatoblastoma
   E. Timing for colectomy determined by polyp burden

9. A 7-year-old boy with mucosal freckling and gynecomastia presents with an intussusception. The lead point was a hamartomatous polyp.
   The management of the child would include all accept
   A. Radical inguinal orchidectomy
   B. Upper GI endoscopy, colonoscopy, and video capsule endoscopy every three years
   C. Elective polypectomy for >1.5 cm polyps
   D. Genetic testing
   E. Aromatase inhibitor therapy

3.5 Rhabdomyosarcoma

1. An 8-year-old boy presents with urinary retention, and several attempts to remove the catheter have failed. The cystoscopic assessment was normal. An MRI scan was performed, which showed prostatic enlargement and no lymphadenopathy seen on the PET scan. Percutaneous or transrectal core needle biopsy showed embryonal rhabdomyosarcoma.
   The management strategy should include all of the following except
   A. Neoadjuvant chemotherapy
   B. Testicular transposition
   C. Conservative surgery
   D. Brachytherapy
   E. Retroperitoneal lymph node dissection

2. A neonate was born with vaginal sarcoma botryoides confirmed on histology after polypectomy
   Management of this baby should include
   A. Lymph node sampling
   B. External beam radiotherapy
   C. Vincristine
   D. Partial vaginectomy
   E. Pelvic CT

3. A 12-year-old boy presents with a right scrotal swelling. MRI showed a 5 cm paratesticular mass. There was no retroperitoneal lymphadenopathy on MRI or PET scan. Therefore, primary radical inguinal orchidectomy was performed. Histology reveals fusion-positive rhabdomyosarcoma and tumour extension beyond tunica vaginalis.
   The management strategy includes all of the following except
   A. Right retroperitoneal lymph node dissection
   B. Radiotherapy
   C. hemi-scrotectomy
   D. Testicular transposition
   E. Chemotherapy

4. A 4-year-old boy presents with a soft tissue lump in his right forearm. There are no clinically palpable axillary lymph nodes. MRI suggests that the mass is localised in the superficial volar compartment. Excision biopsy reveals multiple small, round, blue cells that are positive for desmin and myoglobin. Biopsy also suggests microscopic residual disease on one side.
   The next step in the management of this child is
   A. Pretreatment re-excision
   B. External beam radiotherapy
   C. Chemotherapy
   D. Axillary node dissection
   E. intra-operative radiotherapy

5. A 4-year-old boy presents with fusion-positive rhabdomyosarcoma in his right forearm. R0 resection was achieved, and sentinel node sampling is N0.
   Further treatment in this child includes
   A. No further treatment needed
   B. Radiotherapy
   C. Ray amputation
   D. Doxorubicin
   E. MRI Brain

3.6 Extragonadal Germ Cell Tumours

1. A 9-month-old presented with abdominal distension and constipation. A plain abdominal x-ray showed deformity of the sacrum, and the MRI is displayed

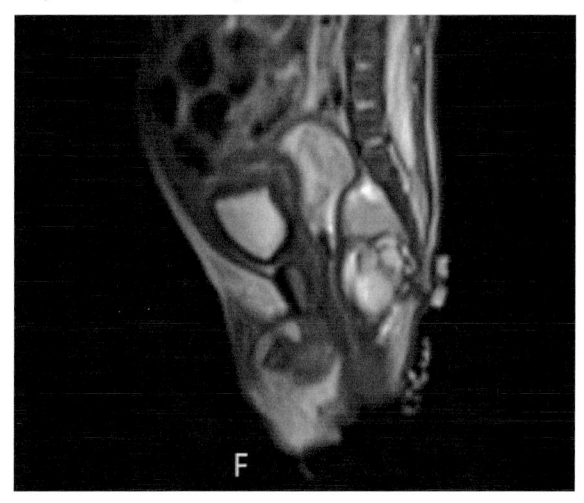

   The management of this baby would include
   A. Anal dilatation
   B. PSARP
   C. Perineal surgery
   D. Abdominoperineal surgery
   E. Neurosurgery

2. A 4-year-old child presents with worsening constipation. On examination, a posterior sagittal bulge was observed displacing the anus anteriorly. MRI showed a sizeable presacral mass. The AFP was 453,173 ng/mL.
   The next step in the management of this child is
   A. Biopsy
   B. Chemotherapy
   C. Tumour resection
   D. Bone marrow aspirate
   E. Brain MRI

3. A baby with a prenatally diagnosed Altman type I sacrococcygeal tumour had a successful resection. Histology confirms a complete resection of a mature teratoma.
   Your follow-up strategy should include all except
   A. Rectal examination
   B. AFP
   C. CA125
   D. CEA
   E. Abdominal US

4. A 10-year-old child presented to the hospital with cough and respiratory distress. Initial CXR prompted the subsequent chest CT as displayed.

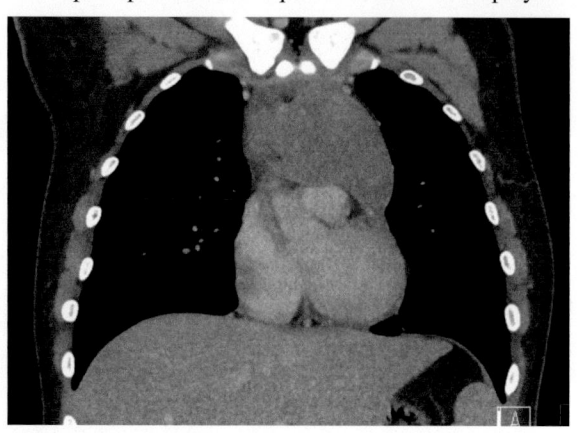

   The management of the child should include all except
   A. Karyotyping
   B. Biopsy
   C. Chemotherapy
   D. Resection
   E. Brain MRI

5. A 9-month-old baby presented to the clinic with gradually increasing abdominal swelling. An X-ray was obtained, and it showed a mass containing tiny bones. The treatment for this baby is
   A. Primary resection
   B. Chemotherapy
   C. Angioembolisation
   D. Sclerotherapy
   E. Radiotherapy

6. A 3-year-old boy was having chemotherapy for retroperitoneal metastasis from a testicular yolk sac tumour. The AFP has returned to normal, but the retroperitoneal mass continued to proliferate. There is no uptake seen on the FDG PET scan. The treatment of this child is
   A. Surgical removal
   B. Change of chemotherapy
   C. Radiotherapy
   D. Angioembolism
   E. Immunotherapy

3.7 Ovarian Tumours

1. A baby girl was prenatally diagnosed to have a pelvic cyst. The postnatal US showed a Left ovarian simple cyst of 70 mm in diameter. She is asymptomatic. The management of the baby would be
   A. US in 3 months
   B. Laparoscopic cystectomy
   C. Oophorectomy
   D. MRI pelvis
   E. HCG, AFP
2. A 12-year-old girl had US for ongoing lower abdominal pain, which showed a 5 cm complex multilocular ovarian mass.
   The management of this child would include all accept
   A. Tumour markers
   B. Serial US
   C. Laparoscopic Cystectomy
   D. MRI
   E. Oophorectomy
3. A 10-year-old girl presented to the emergency department with acute Right iliac fossa pain. A black necrotic torted ovary with a 5 cm cyst containing haemorrhagic fluid was found on laparoscopy.
   The appropriate management of this child would be
   A. Untwisting the ovary
   B. Untwisting the ovary and draining the cyst
   C. Untwisting the ovary and cystectomy
   D. Untwisting the ovary and deroofing the cyst
   E. Oophorectomy
4. On MRI, a 13-year-old girl presented with a complex 10 cm Left ovarian mass have mild ascites. In addition, her AFP, HCG, and CA 125 are all significantly elevated. During salpingo-oophorectomy, you should perform all of the following except
   A. collection ascitic fluid
   B. Iliac node sampling
   C. Omental biopsy
   D. Biopsy of the contralateral ovary
   E. Resection of peritoneal deposits

5. A 10-year-old girl with precocious puberty and hypothyroidism was diagnosed to have a large multiseptated ovarian cyst
   The treatment of the ovarian cyst is
   A. Thyroid hormone replacement
   B. Ovarian sparing cystectomy
   C. Cyst aspiration
   D. Chemotherapy
   E. Oophorectomy

6. A Tumour marker assay in a child with an ovarian tumour showed elevated AFP, HCG and CA125; however, Inhibin was normal.
   The tumour is most likely to be
   A. Dysgerminoma
   B. Immature teratoma
   C. Mucinous carcinoma
   D. Embryonal carcinoma
   E. Sertoli-Leydig cell tumor

7. A 5-year-old girl presented with Isosexual pseudoprecocious puberty and was diagnosed with the most common type of functioning ovarian neoplasm
   In this child, you expect all of the following except
   A. Gonadotropin is low
   B. HCG is high
   C. Inhibin is high
   D. Anti-Mullerian hormone (AMH) is high
   E. Urinary estrogen is high

8. A 10-year-old girl has a solid ovarian tumour. She also had melanocytic nevus on her face and multiple skin pits on her palm and soles.
   All the following statements about her are true except
   A. CA125 and Inhibin are elevated
   B. High risk of basal cell carcinoma
   C. High risk of medulloblastoma
   D. Cerebral calcifications seen
   E. Salpingoophorectomy indicated

9. An 11-year-old girl presented with hirsutism, clitoral hypertrophy, deepening of the voice, and accelerated somatic growth. An ovarian tumour was found during the investigation
   In this child, you would expect
   A. Raised serum testosterone
   B. Raised HCG
   C. Raised gonadotrophin
   D. Low urinary 17-ketosteroids
   E. Raised urinary pregnanetriol

3.8 Testicular Tumours 23

10. On imaging, an 11-year-old girl was diagnosed with a mature cystic teratoma and underwent an ovarian sparing surgery. Multiple 1–3 mm grey nodules are seen on the omentum and pelvic peritoneum during the procedure.
    The management of the lesions is
    A. Biopsy only
    B. Excision of lesions
    C. Cautery of lesions
    D. Chemotherapy
    E. Radiotherapy
11. A phenotypic 15-year-old girl investigated for primary amenorrhea was found to have a 46XY karyotype.
    Due to the risk of development of a particular gonadal neoplasm, it is recommended to perform
    A. Immediate bilateral gonadectomy
    B. Gonadectomy after puberty but before 20 years
    C. Serial US monitoring
    D. Serial tumour marker monitoring
    E. MRI pelvis

3.8 Testicular Tumours

1. A 14-year-old child presents with an insidious, painless Right testicular lump. AFP is normal. The US showed a non-vascular, well-marginated intratesticular mass with a lamellated "onion skin" appearance with alternating hyperechoic and hypoechoic rings.
   The most appropriate treatment for this child is
   A. Inguinal radical orchidectomy
   B. Inguinal testicular sparing surgery with frozen section
   C. Scrotal testicular sparing surgery with frozen section
   D. Inguinal orchidectomy with ipsilateral retroperitoneal lymph node sampling
   E. Serial US monitoring
2. An 18-month old baby had a Right radical inguinal orchidectomy for a testicular tumour and raised AFP. Histology showed Schiller–Duval bodies. There is a residual scrotal disease on histology, but no retroperitoneal lymph nodes were detected on imaging.
   Further management of this child would include all of the following except
   A. 4 Cycles of JEB chemotherapy
   B. Scrotal radiotherapy
   C. Follow-up with serial CXR
   D. Follow-up with serial AFP
   E. Follow-up with serial cross-sectional imaging

3. An 8-year old child has a testicular tumour typically associated with Reinke crystals on histology
   In this child, you are expected to find all except
   A. Precocious puberty
   B. Gynaecomastia
   C. Raised HCG
   D. Raised testosterone
   E. Low luteinizing hormone (LH)
4. A 14-year old boy with an undiagnosed right intraabdominal testis presented with a mass with ascites and retroperitoneal lymph node involvement. Laparotomy was performed to remove the tumour, which was reported to be the most common type of testicular cancer associated with undescended testis.
   Further management of this child would involve
   A. 4 cycles of JEB chemotherapy
   B. 6 cycles of JEB chemotherapy
   C. Retroperitoneal radiotherapy
   D. Retroperitoneal lymph node sampling
   E. Retroperitoneal lymph node dissection
5. An 11-year-old boy with ongoing vague Left testicular pain had the scrotal US. He has no history of undescended testis or previous germ cell tumours, and there is no testicular hypotrophy on examination. [Case courtesy of Dr Naqibullah Foladi, Radiopaedia.org, rID: 83814]

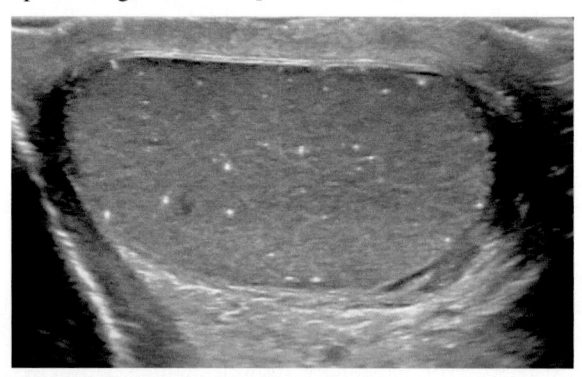

   The management of this child during paediatric age would involve
   A. No further investigation or follow-up
   B. Monthly self-examination from puberty
   C. Annual follow-up with ultrasound
   D. Testicular biopsy
   E. Left orchidectomy

3.9 Adrenal Tumours

1. An 11-year-old girl presents with headaches, fever, palpitations, sweating, weight loss, and sustained hypertension. MIBG SPECT CT is Displayed.

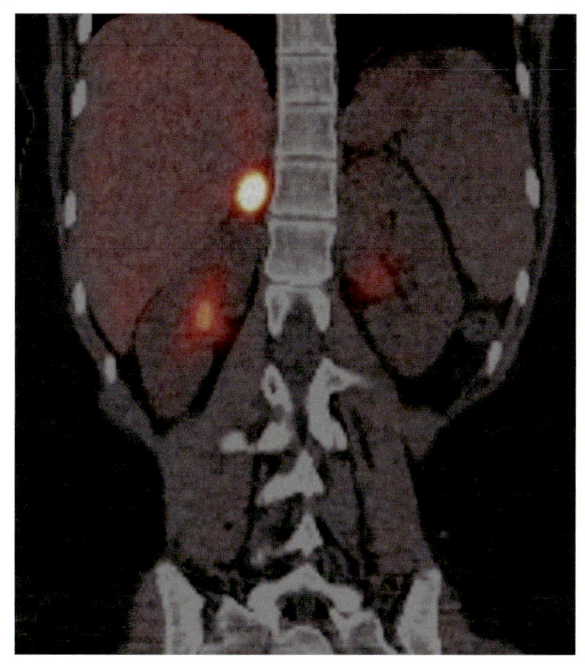

   The next step in management is
   A. Biopsy
   B. Bisoprolol
   C. Corticosteroids
   D. MIBG therapy
   E. Phenoxybenzamine

2. Pheochromocytoma is frequently associated with genetic disorders.
   In children with MEN 2A and pheochromocytoma, all of the following are expected except
   A. Increased metanephrine
   B. Family History
   C. Multicentric
   D. Extra-adrenal site
   E. Hyperparathyroidism

3. Children with Von Hippel-Lindau (VHL) disease have a high risk of developing pheochromocytoma.
   In those children, you would observe all of the following except
   A. Increased metanephrine
   B. Increased normetanephrine
   C. Cerebellar hemangioblastoma
   D. Renal cell carcinoma
   E. Family history

4. A 5-year-old girl presents with hypercortisolism. 24-hour urinary free cortisol was 224 µg/day, and ACTH was 2 ng/L. Cross-sectional imaging of the adrenals showed no mass.
   The most appropriate treatment of this child would be
   A. Unilateral adrenalectomy
   B. Bilateral adrenalectomy
   C. Transsphenoidal hypophysectomy
   D. Mifepristone
   E. corticotrophin-inhibiting peptide

5. A teenage girl presented with hypercortisolism, and her ACTH was 524 ng/L (↑↑). She also had a history of cough, haemoptysis and recurrent pneumonia. In addition, 5-hydroxyindoleacetic acid (5-HIAA) was significantly raised. A mass in the middle lobe of the right lung was identified with no hilar lymph node enlargement.
   The most appropriate treatment of this child would be
   A. Lung parenchymal sparing tumour resection
   B. Right middle lobectomy and lymph node dissection
   C. Right pneumonectomy
   D. Bilateral adrenalectomy
   E. Chest radiotherapy

6. In a child with primary hyperaldosteronism, no aldosteronoma was identified on imaging. Instead, there was a diffuse bilateral adrenocortical hyperplasia.
   The most appropriate treatment is
   A. Unilateral adrenalectomy
   B. Bilateral adrenalectomy
   C. Spironolactone
   D. Radiofrequency ablation
   E. Mifepristone

7. A premature newborn was diagnosed with a hyperechoic Right adrenal on a US scan. Urinary catecholamine metabolites are normal. However, on a repeat scan, the lesion became more hypoechoic.
   The most appropriate management for this baby is
   A. Serial US scans
   B. Cross-sectional imaging
   C. Surgical excision
   D. Radiofrequency ablation
   E. MIBG scan

3.10 Tumours of the Lung and Chest Wall 27

8. A 4-year-old girl who recently migrated from south Brazil presented with features of virilisation and Cushing's syndrome. Genetic analysis showed mutations in the p53 tumour suppressor gene. In addition, DHEA-S and 17-ketosteroids are elevated. Management of this child would include all except
   A. MRI
   B. Resection
   C. Mitotane
   D. Radiotherapy
   E. Iodocholesterol scan

3.10 Tumours of the Lung and Chest Wall

1. A 10-year-old boy had completed his radical therapy for osteosarcoma of the femur but is left with 4 metastatic lung nodules with no other metastases.
   The treatment for the pulmonary nodules is
   A. Chemotherapy
   B. Immunotherapy
   C. Lobectomy
   D. Metastasectomy
   E. Pneumonectomy

2. A 13-year-old boy presents with typical features of an aneurysmal bone cyst of his right fourth rib. It is 4 × 5 cm in diameter and is destroying the nearby tissues.
   The treatment of choice is
   A. Complete surgical excision
   B. Conservative management
   C. Radiotherapy
   D. Chemotherapy
   E. Aspiration

3. A 12-year-old boy presented haematemesis and chest pain, and a CT scan was performed. This tumour is a part of a triad that constitutes a rare syndrome.
   [Case courtesy of Dr Yi-Jin Kuok, Radiopaedia.org, rID: 17407]
   In this child, you would also expect all of the above except
   A. Gastric GIST
   B. Secretary paraganglioma
   C. SDHB mutation
   D. Pheochromocytoma
   E. Hypertension

4. A 9-year old boy with a long history of cough and wheeze was diagnosed with a lung mass. In addition, his 24-hour urinary 5-hydroxyindoleactic acid (5-HIAA) is elevated.
   This child could also have
   A. Hyperthyroidism
   B. Hyperparathyroidism
   C. Cushing's syndrome
   D. Addison's Disease
   E. Hypoaldosteronism

5. A 4-year-old child was treated for suspected pneumonia. A CT was performed when there was no clinical improvement with antibiotics.

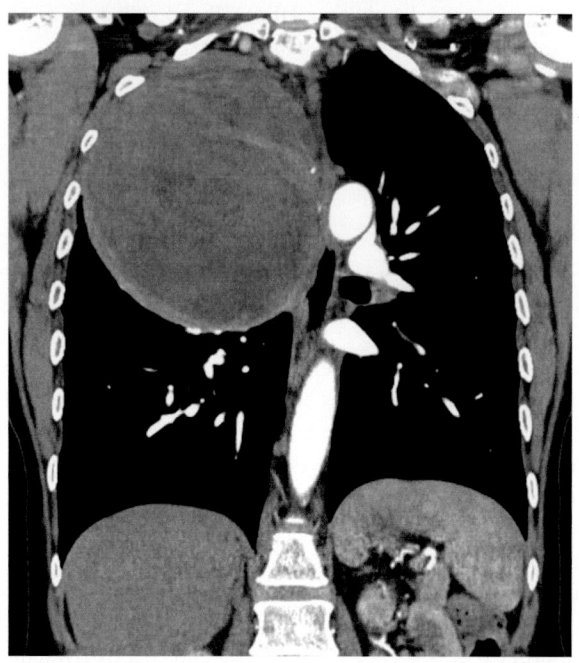

   Your approach to managing this child would be
   A. Primary surgical excision
   B. Biopsy, chemotherapy, then surgery
   C. high dose chemotherapy and stem cell transplantation
   D. Radiotherapy
   E. Embolisation

6. The most appropriate treatment for pulmonary metastasis from Wilm's tumour is?
   A. Metastatectomy
   B. Lobectomy
   C. Chemotherapy
   D. Radiotherapy
   E. Immunotherapy

Head and Neck

4

Anindya Niyogi and Ashok Daya Ram

4.1 Craniofacial Anomalies

1. A 21-year-old lady is undergoing a second-trimester scan for her first pregnancy. She has features of acrocephaly, prominent forehead, hypertelorism, proptosis, broad nasal root, webbed neck, pectus excavatum, cutaneous syndactyly of both hands, total syndactyly of toes of both feet. She mentions that her sister has the same features.
   The antenatal scan should particularly look out for
   A. Spina Bifida
   B. Cervical swellings
   C. Anterior abdominal wall defects
   D. Craniosynostosis and syndactyly
   E. Micrognathia
2. A one-month-old baby is diagnosed to have craniosynostosis.
   The best management would be:
   A. Regular follow up
   B. Regular aspiration
   C. surgical calvarial vault remodelling
   D. Ventriculoatrial shunt
   E. Ventriculoperitoneal shunt

3. A newborn baby boy is diagnosed to have craniosynostosis.
   The best age for surgery is:
   A. Immediate postnatal
   B. 3–9 months
   C. 1–2 years
   D. 5–10 years
   E. After puberty
4. A 6-month-old baby with a restrictive tongue-tie is successfully bottle feeding and gaining weight. However, the mother is worried about future speech development. Your management approach will be
   A. Offer tongue-tie division in the clinic
   B. Offer tongue-tie division under anaesthetic
   C. Assure that tongue-tie will not cause speech problems
   D. Divide tongue-tie in future of the child develops a lisp
   E. Refer to speech and language therapist
5. A 6-month-old baby with Beckwith–Wiedemann syndrome develops obstructive sleep apnoea
   The most appropriate management for the child is
   A. CPAP
   B. Adenoidectomy
   C. Nasal steroids
   D. Tongue reduction surgery
   E. Oral appliances

4.2   Salivary Glands

1. A four-year-old girl presents with a bluish cystic mass on the floor of the mouth, which extends into the right neck. She has developed obstructive sleep apnoea and failure to thrive. MRI confirms a plunging ranula.
   The best management would be:
   A. Sclerotherapy using OK432
   B. Aspiration
   C. Excision of the ranula and the sublingual gland
   D. Excision of the ranula
   E. Conservative management
2. A three-month-old child presents with left-sided soft non-tender parotid swelling with a few associated pigmented cutaneous lesions. The ultrasound demonstrates lobulated hypervascular mass, with arterial and venous signals visible on colour-flow Doppler. She is asymptomatic.
   The next step in the management is:
   A. Conservative management with regular follow up
   B. Superficial parotidectomy
   C. Total parotidectomy
   D. Corticosteroids
   E. Interferon

3. A 10-year-old boy is suspected of having pleomorphic adenoma of the right parotid gland.
   The imaging of choice for the planned excision is:
   A. Plain CT scan
   B. Contrast CT scan
   C. PET scan
   D. Ultrasound scan
   E. MRI scan
4. A 10-year-old boy presents with a rubbery lump over the right parotid gland. MRI suggests a heterogenous confined within the superficial lobe of the parotid. Biopsy revealed the most common nonvascular salivary gland tumour.
   The most appropriate treatment is
   A. Serial MRI follow-up
   B. Superficial parotidectomy
   C. Total parotidectomy
   D. Radical parotidectomy
   E. Extended radical parotidectomy

4.3 Lymph Node Disorders

1. A four-year-old boy acutely develops extensive nonsuppurative, nontender cervical lymphadenopathy associated with dry red cracked lips, red swollen tongue, erythema of mouth, and pharynx red eyes.
   The management of this patient is
   A. Incision and drainage of cervical lymph node abscesses
   B. Excision of all affected lymph nodes
   C. Conservative management with bed rest and analgesics
   D. Intravenous immunoglobulins and Aspirin
   E. Broad-spectrum antibiotics
2. A one-year-old boy presents with a 2-week history of right-sided supraclavicular lymph node enlargement. No treatment has been given previously.
   The next step in the management is:
   A. Antibiotics for four weeks
   B. Excisional biopsy
   C. Incisional Biopsy
   D. FNAC
   E. CT of the neck

3. A three-year-old girl develops rapid onset of unilateral left-sided submandibular lymph node enlargement, which is minimally tender, firm and rubbery and well circumscribed. She has not responded to first-line antibiotics. She has no signs of systemic illness, and the chest X-ray is normal. It has been present for seven weeks. The treatment of choice is:
   A. Second-line antibiotics
   B. Excision of the affected lymph node
   C. Incision and drainage
   D. Aspiration
   E. Continue conservative management
4. A four-year-old boy is scheduled to have an excisional biopsy for right-sided cervical lymphadenopathy.
   The pre-operative investigation must include
   A. Ultrasound of the neck, axilla and groin
   B. Ultrasound of the liver and spleen
   C. MRI of the neck
   D. PET scan
   E. Chest X-ray

4.4 Thyroid and Parathyroid glands

1. A solid mass is encountered during the procedure to excise a thyroglossal cyst. The next step would be to:
   A. Excise the mass in total and continue with the Sistrunk procedure
   B. Send a specimen for a frozen section before proceeding accordingly
   C. On table ultrasound to recheck the mass and the thyroid gland
   D. Abandon the procedure, close the incision and investigate thoroughly
   E. Incisional biopsy and close the incision
2. A 12-year-old girl is incidentally found to have papillary carcinoma of the thyroid gland during the Sistrunk procedure for a thyroglossal cyst. There was capsular invasion and lymph node enlargement.
   The next step in the management is:
   A. Regular follow up
   B. Radioactive iodine ablation
   C. Completion thyroidectomy, nodal dissection, and radioiodine ablation
   D. Completion thyroidectomy and nodal dissection
   E. Radiotherapy
3. A normal parathyroid gland has been devascularised during thyroidectomy.
   The next step in the management is:
   A. Excision of the affected gland
   B. Microvascular surgery to restore blood supply
   C. No intervention
   D. Removal of all 4 glands
   E. Autotransplantation into the sternocleidomastoid

4.5 Neck Cysts and Sinuses   33

4. A child presents with tertiary hyperparathyroidism secondary to end-stage renal failure. Medical therapy for the condition has failed.
   The best surgical option for the condition is
   A. Resection of visibly enlarged parathyroid glands
   B. Three and a Half gland parathyroidectomy
   C. Hemithyroidectomy with ipsilateral parathyroid gland removal
   D. Total parathyroidectomy with autotransplantation
   E. Unilateral parathyroidectomy
5. A baby is diagnosed to have MEN IIB syndrome.
   The most appropriate management of the child's thyroid gland is
   A. Prophylactic total thyroidectomy
   B. Prophylactic subtotal thyroidectomy
   C. Prophylactic hemithyroidectomy
   D. Diagnostic FNAB and proceed
   E. Regular MRI scans and proceed
6. A 12-year-old child presented with a solitary thyroid nodule, and her TSH level was low. Thyroid scintigraphy demonstrated increased uptake within the nodule is consistent with an autonomous nodular function.
   The most appropriate management is
   A. US-guided FNAC
   B. Repeat the US in 6 months
   C. Ipsilateral lobectomy
   D. Total thyroidectomy
   E. Levothyroxine

4.5 Neck Cysts and Sinuses

1. A second-trimester foetus is diagnosed with cervical teratoma on ultrasound, confirmed by the MRI.
   In planning the delivery of the foetus:
   A. Preterm delivery is recommended
   B. Normal vaginal delivery at term is advocated
   C. Delivery at the ECMO centre is recommended
   D. C section delivery at the tertiary centre is recommended
   E. EXIT procedure is recommended in all foetuses
2. A one-year-old boy has a first branchial cleft anomaly and has an extreme risk of anaesthesia. The fistula is causing persistent discharge, which is occasionally purulent.
   The next step in the management is:
   A. Ethanol ablation
   B. High-risk surgery
   C. Conservative management
   D. Radio ablation
   E. Chemo ablation

3. A six-year-old presents with a left-sided anterior triangle cystic lesion that enlarges with Valsalva manoeuvre.
   The management is
   A. Conservative management
   B. Complete surgical excision
   C. Aspiration
   D. Sclerotherapy
   E. Radiotherapy
4. During surgical excision in the neck near the hyoid bone, diagnostic doubt exists between thyroglossal duct cyst and dermoid cyst.
   The best course of action is
   A. Excise the visible cyst
   B. Biopsy and proceed
   C. On table ultrasound
   D. Formal Sistrunk procedure
   E. Abandon the procedure till further investigations
5. A child presents with a longitudinal area of atrophic skin along the anterior midline of the neck. There is a skin tag at the upper end and small sinus tracts at the inferior aspect. Secretions are noted in the cleft.
   The best management is
   A. Early surgical excision
   B. Excision of the skin tag
   C. Excision of the sinus tracts
   D. Conservative management
   E. Physiotherapy

Thorax

5

Anindya Niyogi and Ashok Daya Ram

5.1 Disorders of the Breast

1. A 15-year-old boy presents to the clinic with bilateral gynaecomastia. Which drug is the potential cause:
   A. Rifampicin
   B. Thyroxine
   C. Propranolol
   D. Tricyclic Antidepressants
   E. Furosemide
2. A teenage boy presents to the surgical clinic with bilateral gynaecomastia. Examination of the testes is essential to rule out:
   A. Klinefelter's syndrome
   B. Down's syndrome
   C. Patau syndrome
   D. Prada Willi syndrome
   E. Di George syndrome

A. Niyogi (✉)
King's College Hospital, London, UK

A. D. Ram
Norfolk and Norwich University Hospital, Norwich, UK

© The Author(s), under exclusive license to Springer Nature Switzerland AG 2025
A. Niyogi, A. D. Ram, *MCQs in Paediatric Surgery*,
https://doi.org/10.1007/978-3-031-94124-5_5

3. A 14-year-old boy presents with bilateral gynaecomastia, increased belly fat, tall stature with longer legs and a shorter torso. He also has delayed puberty. In addition, there is less muscle and facial hair compared to peers, small penis, small firm testicles, low energy levels and weak bones.
   The genetics test will most likely reveal:
   A. XYY
   B. XXY
   C. XXX
   D. XXXY
   E. X0
4. A 15-year-old girl presents with a slowly growing painless lump in the upper outer quadrant of her right breast. A well-defined hypoechoic nodule measuring 4.5 × 4.0 × 3.0 cm was found on ultrasound. Core biopsy showed tumour cells with vacuolated, foamy cytoplasm and large intracellular and extracellular pale blue to thick pink secretions.
   The best treatment is:
   A. Surgical excision only
   B. Surgical excision followed by local radiotherapy
   C. Neoadjuvant chemotherapy
   D. Adjuvant chemotherapy
   E. Localised radiotherapy
5. A 15-year-old girl presents with a right breast lump. Ultrasound showed an ill-defined mass composed of multiple small cysts resembling swiss cheese.
   The treatment is:
   A. Right mastectomy
   B. Adjuvant chemotherapy
   C. Wide surgical excision
   D. Conservative management
   E. Neoadjuvant chemotherapy
6. A 15-year-old child presents with rapidly growing bilateral breast lumps. She was born with exomphalos and hypoglycemia.
   The most appropriate treatment is
   A. Observation
   B. Wide local excision
   C. Mastectomy
   D. Neoadjuvant chemotherapy
   E. Tamoxifen
7. A 14-year-old girl presents with galactorrhoea, and an MRI brain showed a pituitary mass.
   The initial treatment is
   A. Dienogest
   B. Mifepristone
   C. Cabergoline
   D. Surgery
   E. Estradiol

5.2 Congenital Chest Wall Deformities   37

8. In a teenage girl of Ashkenazi Jewish heritage with a family history of early-onset breast cancers, molecular genetic testing confirms an inherited cancer-predisposition syndrome
   All of the following treatment options have some role in this syndrome, except
   A. Prophylactic mastectomy
   B. Tamoxifen
   C. Levonorgestrel
   D. Talazoparib
   E. Risk-reducing salpingo-oophorectomy

9. A 6-year-old girl presents with isolated bilateral symmetrical breast development with no other secondary sexual characteristics
   The best management is
   A. Expectant management
   B. Tamoxifen
   C. Full endocrine workup
   D. Mammogram
   E. Genetic testing

10. A 6-day old neonate develops an isolated right-sided breast abscess
    The most common causative organism is sensitive to the antibiotic, which works in the following mechanism
    A. Inhibition of Folic acid synthesis
    B. Inhibition of Cell wall synthesis
    C. Inhibition of DNA synthesis
    D. Inhibition of 30S subunit of ribosome
    E. Inhibition of 50S subunit of ribosome

5.2 Congenital Chest Wall Deformities

1. A one-month-old boy with mild respiratory distress was found to have paradoxical respiration, a narrow chest, missing ribs on both sides with only 7 ribs on either side, micrognathia, cleft palate and hearing loss.
   The next step in the management of this patient is:
   A. Gastrostomy
   B. Tracheostomy
   C. Repair of the chest wall
   D. Involve palliative care team
   E. Repair of cleft palate

2. Post-mortem examination of the baby who died of respiratory distress found the features of e multiple alternating hemivertebrae affecting all the thoracic and lumbar spine, multiple posterior fusion of ribs, short neck and thorax, protruding abdomen with an umbilical hernia, right atrial appendage and a duplex urinary system. A pre-mortal X-ray in the NICU demonstrated a crab-like appearance in the rib cage. Parents are phenotypically normal, and there is no other family history.
   In counselling the parents for subsequent offspring having the same condition
   A. 75% chance of having affected baby
   B. 50% chance of having affected baby
   C. 50% chance of the baby being a carrier
   D. 25% chance of having affected baby
   E. 25% chance the baby being a carrier
3. A 9-month-old boy has needed intermittent hospital admissions for respiratory support and has been diagnosed with Asphyxiating thoracic dystrophy.
   The usual long-term respiratory outcome of this patient is
   A. Improvement after one year of age
   B. Ongoing deterioration
   C. Invariably fatal within 3 years
   D. Unpredictable
   E. Unchanged
4. A newborn baby boy is seen to have a superior partial bifid sternum.
   Which of the following is associated with
   A. Ectopic heart
   B. Skin defect
   C. Intact pericardium
   D. Cardiac defects
   E. Diaphragmatic hernia
5. A 14-year-old girl has got absent unilateral anterior axillary fold and syndactyly of the right hand.
   Which of the following physical findings is present
   A. Hypertrophy of the breast
   B. Accessory nipples
   C. Winged scapula
   D. Excessive axillary hair
   E. Hypolucent lung
6. A patient with pectus excavatum is counselled for suction vacuum bell therapy. The following condition is a contraindication for him.
   A. Haller index of greater than 3
   B. Marfan's syndrome
   C. Osteogenesis imperfecta
   D. Less than 14 years of age
   E. Female gender

5.3 Congenital Diaphragmatic Hernia and Eventration   39

7. A 13-year-old boy is being planned for a Nuss procedure for pectus excavatum. His parents said he is prone to allergies.
   The following allergy test is indicated.
   A. Chromium
   B. Iron
   C. Titanium
   D. Nickel
   E. Aluminium
8. In a child undergoing the Ravitch procedure, the following measure is observed to prevent asphyxiating thoracic dystrophy.
   A. Avoiding the procedure before 12 years of age
   B. Removing 8 pairs of costal cartilages
   C. leaving a few millimetres of cartilage on the rib
   D. Removal of all cartilage on the sternal end
   E. Removal of the xiphoid process

5.3 Congenital Diaphragmatic Hernia and Eventration

1. A 14-year-old girl presenting with intermittent left upper quadrant abdominal pain was diagnosed on a CT scan to have a large left-sided sub-diaphragmatic splenic cyst. During the laparoscopy to remove the cyst, the spleen was normal. A cyst is still visible in the left upper quadrant.
   The most likely diagnosis is
   A. Ruptured splenic cyst
   B. Left-sided pneumonia
   C. Hydatic cyst of the left lobe of the liver
   D. Epidermoid cyst of the diaphragm
   E. Gastric duplication
2. A three-week-old boy born at 30 weeks is found to have bilateral diaphragmatic eventration and is still needing ventilatory support.
   The next step in the management is
   A. Continue conservative management
   B. Unilateral abdominal plication
   C. Unilateral Thoracoscopic plication
   D. Bilateral thoracoscopic diaphragmatic plication
   E. Bilateral abdominal diaphragmatic plication
3. An 8-year-old girl with Rett syndrome presenting with recurrent pneumonia was found to have left-sided diaphragmatic eventration.
   The next step in the management is:
   A. Conservative management
   B. Non-invasive ventilation
   C. Mechanical ventilation
   D. Thoracoscopic plication of the diaphragm
   E. Intrinsic diaphragmatic muscle stimulation

4. A 6-month-old boy with left-sided diaphragmatic eventration presents with intractable non-bilious vomiting.
   The next step in the management is
   A. Ultrasound scan
   B. Thoracoscopy
   C. Upper GI contrast study
   D. Anti emetics
   E. Lateral Chest X-ray
5. A 1-year-old boy with Down's syndrome had a chest X-ray for suspected pneumonia

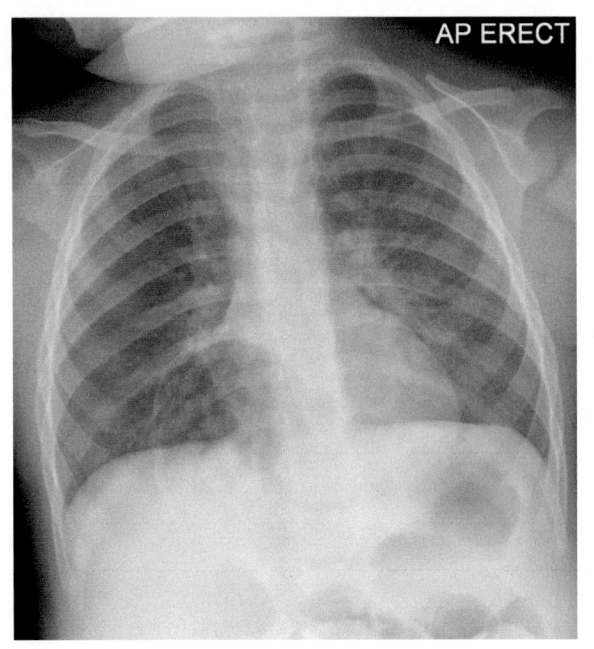

   During surgical repair, the following is observed
   A. The sac is never present
   B. The sac must always be excised
   C. The sac can be left alone if adherent to pericardium
   D. The sac is inverted
   E. The sac is included in the suture of the defect.
6. A 28-week pregnant lady has a fetus with a congenital diaphragmatic hernia on the left side with no other major structural or chromosomal defects. Observed-to-expected lung-to-head ratio is 24%.
   The most appropriate management is
   A. Early induction of labour
   B. Fetal repair
   C. Fetoscopic endotracheal occlusion
   D. Maternal steroid
   E. Termination

5.4 Congenital Lung Malformations 41

7. The echocardiogram of a baby with left CDH showed right ventricular dysfunction, pulmonic and tricuspid valve regurgitation, and right-to-left ductal shunting. The first line of treatment is
   A. Extracorporeal membrane oxygenation
   B. High Frequency Oscillatory ventilation
   C. Inhaled nitric oxide
   D. Milrinone
   E. Sildenafil

5.4 Congenital Lung Malformations

1. A fetus of 26 weeks gestation is found to have Right lower lobe CPAM. The maximum length of the lesion is 18 mm, the maximum height is 13 mm and the maximum width is 22 mm. The head circumference is 242 mm. The appearances are microcystic.
   The next step in the management of the fetus is:
   A. Regular ultrasound scan
   B. Maternal steroids
   C. Fetal steroids
   D. Exit procedure
   E. Fetal surgery
2. An elective left lower lobectomy was performed on a one-year-old boy.
   The following microscopic features distinguish CPAM from normal lung tissue.
   A. Polypoid projections of submucosa
   B. Decreased smooth muscle and elastic tissue within cyst walls
   C. Absence of cartilage
   D. Absence of mucous secreting cells
   E. The presence of inflammation
3. A 26-year-old female underwent an anomaly scan at the 20th week of gestation. The scan demonstrated an echogenic mass occupying the left hemithorax and displacing the heart toward the right. The stomach bubble was normally located. Two cystic lesions of size 3 mm and 4 mm were seen in the apical and basal region of the echogenic mass lesion. Colour Doppler did not reveal any demonstrable flow in this lesion.
   The next investigation is:
   A. Fetal MRI
   B. Chromosomal analysis
   C. Echocardiogram
   D. Repeat ultrasound
   E. Maternal alpha-fetoprotein

4. A follow up ultrasound at 34 weeks of a fetus with CCM volume of 1.6 of a lesion with multiple cysts of 2–4 mm in size also demonstrated features of ascites, pleural effusion and scalp oedema.
   The next step in the management of the fetus is:
   A. Repeat ultrasound in one week
   B. Aspiration
   C. Thoracoamniotic shunt
   D. Steroids
   E. Urgent delivery

5. A baby needs to undergo resection of emphysematous lung tissue secondary to congenital lobar emphysema.
   During the induction of anaesthesia, the agent to avoid is:
   A. Oxygen
   B. Sevoflurane
   C. Nitric Oxide
   D. Halothane
   E. Isoflurane

6. A lobectomy specimen in a 3-month-old boy with congenital lobar emphysema is sent for histology.
   Which feature is found in histology?
   A. The airways are normal in number, size and structure
   B. Evidence of acinar destruction
   C. Evidence of terminal bronchiolar inflammation
   D. Decreased collagen in alveolar basement membrane
   E. The arteries are abnormal in structure

7. A 1-year-old child has left extralobar pulmonary sequestration
   The arterial supply most commonly arises from
   A. Aorta
   B. Coeliac trunk
   C. Gastric
   D. Intercostal arteries
   E. Splenic artery

8. A newborn baby has a large extra lobar sequestration on the left side of the chest.
   The most likely complication if the lesion is not removed is
   A. Recurrent pneumonia
   B. Spontaneous haemorrhage
   C. Left to right shunt
   D. Risk of malignancy
   E. Cardiac failure

9. A follow-up ultrasound scan of a 24-week fetus with left-sided microcystic CCAM demonstrated a CCAM volume ratio of 1.5 with mild features of hydrops. The next step in the management is:
   A. Maternal betamethasone
   B. Serial ultrasound
   C. Thoracoamniotic shunt
   D. Preterm delivery
   E. Fetal surgery

5.5 Oesophageal Rupture and Perforation

1. A 4-year-old boy complains of chest pain 2 h after balloon dilatation of oesophageal stricture.
   Your next step in management is
   A. Chest X ray
   B. Endoscopy
   C. ECG
   D. Upper GI contrast study
   E. PPI

2. During a Foreign body retrieval from the oesophagus of a 12-month-old boy, the anaesthetist noted a sudden increase in ventilatory pressures with no air entry on the right side with left-sided tracheal deviation.
   The next step is:
   A. Chest X ray
   B. Needle thoracocentesis
   C. On table contrast study
   D. Replace ET tube
   E. Thoracotomy

3. After a difficult NG insertion in a one-day-old premature baby, an X-ray was taken, as shown below.

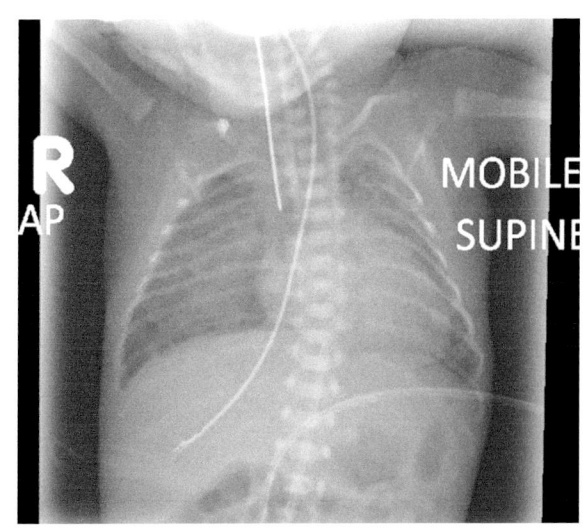

The next step is:
A. TOF/OA repair
B. Remove the tube
C. Water soluble contrast via the NG tube.
D. Advance the NG
E. Endoscopy

4. A teenage boy suddenly develops respiratory distress associated with vomiting, coughing and chest pain. CT Chest is displayed.

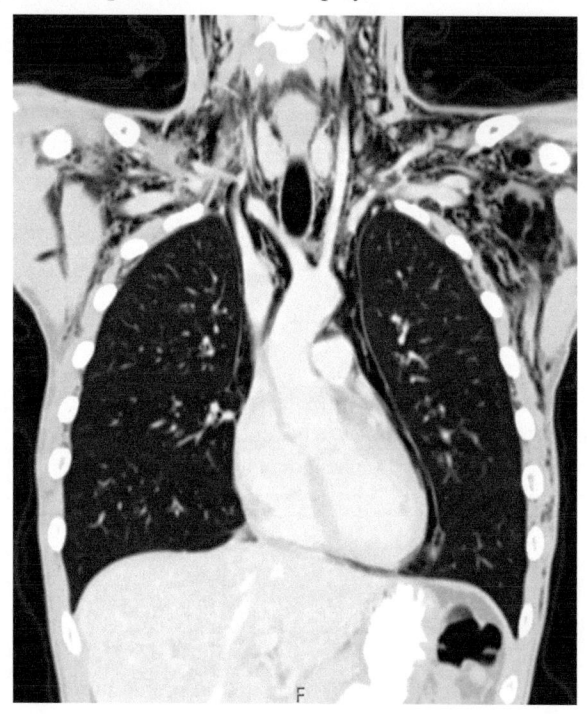

What is the next step
A. NG insertion
B. Upper GI endoscopy
C. Intubation
D. Chest drain insertion
E. Oesophagogram

5. A 6-week-old baby has an ongoing saliva leak in the chest drain after a TOF/OA repair. The baby is being managed with antibiotics and TAT.
   The next step is
   A. Conservative management
   B. Repair of the leak
   C. Oesophagostomy
   D. Gastrostomy
   E. Trans gastric jejunostomy
6. After a difficult removal of a foreign body in a 12-year-old child the day before, she presents with massive hematemesis with hemodynamic instability.
   The most appropriate immediate management is
   A. Observation
   B. Upper GI Endoscopy
   C. CT Thorax
   D. Sengstaken-Blackmore tube
   E. Thoracotomy
7. A seven-year-old child presented with a history of ingestion of a foreign body 3 days ago. Chest X-ray demonstrates a metallic foreign body in the middle oesophagus with right-sided pneumothorax.
   The next step in the management is:
   A. Right thoracotomy
   B. Upper GI contrast study
   C. CT chest
   D. Thoracoscopy
   E. Oesophagoscopic retrieval

5.6 Oesophageal Atresia

1. A one-day-old baby diagnosed with Oesophageal atresia with distal trachea-oesophageal fistula develops respiratory distress with a tense abdomen.
   The best management is:
   A. Occluding the fistula with Fogarty catheter placed via oesophagoscope
   B. Passage of an uncuffed endotracheal tube distal to the fistula, and conventional ventilation
   C. Emergency extra pleural ligation of the tracho oesophageal fistula
   D. Positioning the child, suction and increasing the ventilatory parameters to stabilize the child
   E. Emergency trans pleural ligation of trachea oesophageal fistula

2. A term neonate is born with the antenatal findings of absent stomach bubble and polyhydramnios in the mother. X-ray of the baby is displayed.

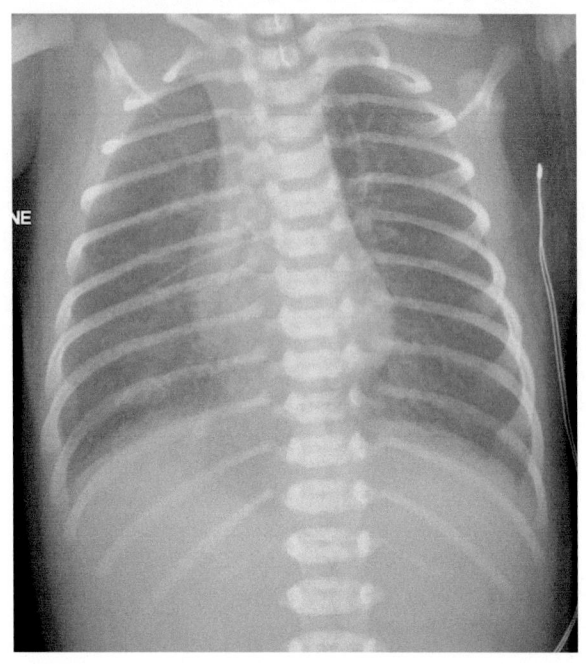

The highest probability of the child having a right sided aortic arch is:
A. Tetralogy of Fallot
B. Dextrocardia with abdominal situs solitus
C. Abdominal situs inversus with levocardia
D. Dextrocardia with polysplenia
E. 13 pairs of ribs

3. A term baby is born with VSD, Choanal atresia, right-sided renal agenesis and a coloboma. The baby cannot feed; thus, an NG was attempted, coiled in the upper oesophagus.
The most likely associated condition the child may have is:
A. Congenital oesophageal stenosis
B. Tracheo-bronchial remnants
C. Tracheal cleft
D. Type C tracheo-oesophageal fistula
E. Type E tracheo-oesophageal fistula

5.6 Oesophageal Atresia

4. A 6-month-old boy had a previous successful repair of OA/TOF, after which the child tolerated milk feeds well. During weaning, the baby presented with dysphagia. Upper GI contrast demonstrated a segmental narrowing just above the gastro-oesophageal junction.
   The next step in the management is:
   A. Balloon dilatation
   B. Resection and anastomosis
   C. Oesophageal myotomy
   D. Antispasmodics
   E. Fundoplication
5. A term neonate with Type C Oesophageal atresia and tracheo oesophageal fistula is planned for theatre the next day. Overnight, the child develops respiratory distress.
   Initial first management is:
   A. Ligation of the fistula
   B. Intubation
   C. Replacing the Replogle tube
   D. Needle decompression of the stomach
   E. Broad spectrum antibiotics
6. A baby with OA/TOF self-ventilating in air develops severe respiratory distress with massive abdominal distension while awaiting surgery.
   The next step in the management is:
   A. Paralysis
   B. Thoracotomy
   C. Intubation
   D. Abdominal X ray
   E. Laparotomy
7. Anastomotic leak after a TOF/OA repair had failed conservative management and thus had a cervical oesophagostomy.
   The subsequent surgical procedure is:
   A. Re anastomosis
   B. Jejunal interposition
   C. Serial lengthening
   D. PTFE graft
   E. Gastrostomy

8. 2 months after successful repair of OA/TOF, the baby develops progressive respiratory symptoms and life-threatening apnoeic spells. Upper GI endoscopy is normal; the impedance study revealed a Boix Ochoa score of 3.
   The next step is:
   A. Aortopexy
   B. Caffeine
   C. Fundoplication
   D. Transgastric jejunal tube
   E. Omeprazole
9. A Collis gastroplasty has been performed to achieve a tension free anastomosis of long gap oesophageal atresia.
   The procedure always requires:
   A. Gastrostomy
   B. Fundoplication
   C. Oesophagostomy
   D. Circular Myotomy
   E. Surgical jejunostomy
10. During the repair of TOF/OA, a distal oesophageal stenosis was noted.
    The most appropriate management is:
    A. Resection and anastomosis of the stenotic segment
    B. Dilatation of the stenosis
    C. Jejunal interposition
    D. Gastrostomy
    E. Oesophagostomy

5.7 Foreign Body Ingestion

1. A toddler was seen to have swallowed a plastic toy piece by parents 8 h ago and thus brought to ED. He is asymptomatic.
   The next course of action is
   A. X ray
   B. Upper GI endoscopy and retrieval
   C. Conservative management
   D. Inform child protection services
   E. Keep nil by mouth
2. A toddler presents with parents giving a history of dysphagia after a food bolus ingestion 6 h earlier. X-ray was unremarkable.
   The next course of action is
   A. Water soluble contrast study
   B. Upper GI endoscopy
   C. CT scan
   D. Repeat X ray in 24 h
   E. Admit and observe

5.7 Foreign Body Ingestion

3. A 2-year-old boy was taken to the theatre to remove a foreign body in the oesophagus ingested 10 days ago. He presented with initial dysphagia, then worsening intermittent hematemesis. The foreign body was found alongside a submucosal hematoma in the oesophagus during endoscopy.
   The next step is:
   A. Abandon the procedure and arrange a CT scan
   B. Carefully remove the foreign body
   C. Biopsy of the submucosal lesion
   D. Push the foreign body into the stomach
   E. Left thoracotomy

4. After a foreign body ingestion, a two-year-old boy has developed an aorto-oesophageal fistula.
   The best surgical approach is:
   A. Left thoracotomy
   B. Right thoracotomy
   C. Thoracoscopy
   D. Abdominal
   E. Upper GI Endoscopic

5. After a traumatic removal of a coin in the middle oesophagus in a one-year-old child, he develops a tracho-oesophageal fistula.
   The best management approach is
   A. Thoracoscopic
   B. Bronchoscopic
   C. Oesophagoscopic
   D. Right thoracotomy
   E. Left thoracotomy

6. A button battery was removed easily via rigid oesophagoscopy 3 h after ingestion, and the child was ready to go home.
   Post discharge management includes:
   A. Contrast study
   B. CT scan
   C. Manometry
   D. pH impedance study
   E. X-ray

7. Parents brought a toddler who had swallowed a metallic toy an hour ago which was found to be in the upper oesophagus on X ray. The child is coughing.
   The next course of action is
   A. Repeat X-ray in 12 h
   B. Immediate retrieval under GA
   C. Encourage coughing
   D. Encourage swallowing
   E. Admit and observe

8. A toddler was brought to the hospital by parents after accidental ingestion of drain cleaner.
   The most appropriate next step for management is
   A. Encourage fluid intake
   B. Endoscopy
   C. NG tube insertion
   D. Intubation
   E. Open gastrostomy

5.8 Gastroesophageal Reflux Disease

1. A 14-year-old was prescribed omeprazole for a hiatus hernia. One year after continuous use of the medicine, the child develops tetany, muscle weakness, and delirium.
   The most likely cause of his symptoms is
   A. Hypocalcemia
   B. Hypomagnesemia
   C. Hypokalemia
   D. Metabolic alkalosis
   E. Respiratory alkalosis

2. A 13-year-old girl takes regular omeprazole for Barrett's oesophagus. She develops depression following a period of domestic abuse that has not responded to cognitive behavioural therapy.
   Which of the following antidepressants requires additional monitoring and adjusted dose?
   A. Trazodone
   B. Amitriptyline
   C. Citalopram
   D. Duloxetine
   E. Mirtazapine

3. A 2-year-old child presented with a long history of non-bilious vomiting. 8 weeks ago, he was started on 15 mg lansoprazole orodispersible tablet once daily. He continued to vomit and had two chest infections.
   The next step in management is
   A. Upper GI contrast
   B. Upper GI endoscopy
   C. pH Multichannel Intraluminal Impedance
   D. Transgastric jejunal tube
   E. Fundoplication

5.8 Gastroesophageal Reflux Disease

4. A 9-year-old girl presents with dysphagia and vomiting, which has not improved after two months of PPI treatment. The endoscopic appearance of the oesophagus is shown [Image courtesy of Samir at the English-language Wikipedia, CC BY-SA 3.0, via Wikimedia Commons]

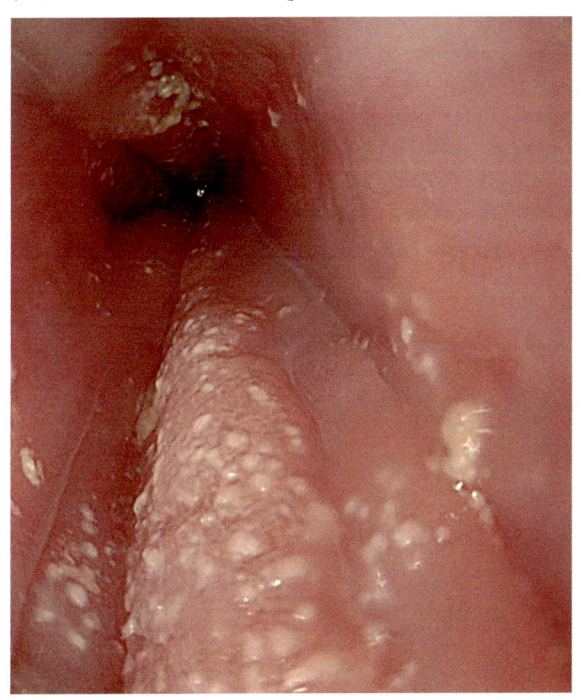

   The next line of treatment is
   A. Topical corticosteroid
   B. Antihistamines
   C. Alginates
   D. Oesophageal dilatation
   E. Fundoplication

5. A 15-year-old boy has Barrett's oesophagus, which extends to 2.5 cm from the gastro-oesophageal junction proximally. Histology confirms intestinal metaplasia but no dysplasia
   He should receive endoscopic surveillance
   A. Never
   B. Every 6 months
   C. Yearly
   D. Every 2–3 years
   E. Every 3–5 years

6. You have decided to perform a partial posterior fundoplication on a 14-year-old boy with a hiatus hernia.
   The procedure is also called
   A. Dor Fundoplication
   B. Thal Fundoplication
   C. Toupet Fundoplication
   D. Watson Fundoplication
   E. Boix-Ochoa Fundoplication
7. A 3-month-old breastfed baby with gastroesophageal reflux is failing to thrive despite maximal pharmacological therapy.
   The next step in the following expressed breast milk additive
   A. Rice cereal
   B. Gelatin
   C. Xanthum gum
   D. Carob bean gum
   E. Pectin

Abdomen

Anindya Niyogi and Ashok Daya Ram

6.1 Congenital Defects of the Abdominal Wall

1. A baby girl is born at 37 weeks with exomphalos and a large tongue.
   The most common chromosomal anomaly associated with her condition is:
   A. Hypomethylation of maternally inherited copy of the IC2 region
   B. Hypomethylation of paternally inherited copy of the IC2 region
   C. Deletion of maternally inherited copy of the IC2 region
   D. Deletion of paternally inherited copy of the IC2 region
   E. Uniparental disomy of the IC2 region
2. The Mother of a baby girl with exomphalos and Beckwith-Wiedemann syndrome tested positive for the genetic mutation of the condition.
   The following procedure will reduce the chances of the next baby inheriting the condition.
   A. Paternal Bone marrow transplant
   B. Preimplantation genetic testing
   C. Fetal gene therapy
   D. Maternal steroids
   E. Exchange transfusion

A. Niyogi (✉)
King's College Hospital, London, UK

A. D. Ram
Norfolk and Norwich University Hospital, Norwich, UK

3. A baby boy is born with exomphalos, anterior diaphragmatic hernia, sternal defect and pericardial defect.
   The most common intra-cardiac defect associated with the condition is:
   A. ASD
   B. VSD
   C. TOF
   D. Pulmonary stenosis
   E. Transposition of great vessels
4. A baby is born with the Pentalogy of Cantrell.
   The most important prognostic factor among the following is:
   A. Size of the exomphalos
   B. Size of the anterior diaphragmatic defect
   C. Location of the ectopic heart
   D. intracardiac defects
   E. Length of sternal defect.
5. On an antenatal scan in a fetus with gastroschisis at 34 weeks of gestation, the diameter of the intraabdominal small intestine was 15 mm.
   The most appropriate management of this pregnancy is
   A. Immediate caesarean section
   B. Immediate induction of labour
   C. Caesarean section at 36 weeks
   D. Induction of labour at 36 weeks
   E. Wait for natural labour
6. During delayed closure of exomphalos in a 2-year-old boy, abdominal wall closure could not be achieved.
   Which of the following would facilitate abdominal closure?
   A. Division of anterior rectus sheath
   B. Division of posterior rectus sheath
   C. Division of external oblique
   D. Rectus muscle flap
   E. Transversus abdominis flap

6.2　Inguinal Hernias and Hydroceles

1. Geigel reflex is generated by cutaneous stimulation of the inner thigh in females
   The efferent fibres of this reflex are carried by
   A. Iliohypogastric nerve
   B. Ilioinguinal nerve
   C. Genital branch of genitofemoral nerve
   D. Femoral branch of genitofemoral nerve
   E. Pudendal nerve

6.2 Inguinal Hernias and Hydroceles

2. While performing an open inguinal herniotomy, you identify a nerve after splitting the external oblique.
   The nerve carries motor fibres to
   A. External oblique
   B. Internal oblique
   C. Cremaster
   D. Pyramidalis
   E. Quadratus lumborum
3. During open herniotomy, you encounter brisk bleeding while dissecting the spermatic cord
   The artery to this region is a branch of
   A. External iliac artery
   B. Inferior epigastric artery
   C. Superficial epigastric artery
   D. Deep external pudendal artery
   E. Deep circumflex iliac artery
4. During laparoscopy for perforated appendicitis in a 12-year-old boy, a right patent processus vaginalis was found
   The next step in management is
   A. Observation
   B. Laparoscopic repair during appendicectomy
   C. Open herniotomy during appendicectomy
   D. Laparoscopic repair on a future date
   E. Open herniotomy on a future date
5. While performing laparoscopic inguinal hernia repair in a 2-year-old boy, bilateral absent vas deferens was noted.
   This child can also have a mutation in a gene located in
   A. The long arm of chromosome 1
   B. The short arm of chromosome 3
   C. The long arm of chromosome 7
   D. The short arm of chromosome 9
   E. The long arm of chromosome 13
6. A 15-year-old boy presents with intermittent right inguinal swelling. He underwent an open appendicectomy five years ago.
   Which of the following surgical technique will have the lowest recurrence
   A. Stoppa
   B. Marcy
   C. Bassini
   D. Lichtenstein
   E. Shouldice

6.3 Undescended Testis

1. baby was born at term with unilateral undescended testis. GP referred you as the testis remained undescended on the 6-week baby check.
   The most appropriate action is
   A. Accept referral for assessment
   B. Assess baby at 3 months of age
   C. Request reassessment by GP at 5 months
   D. Assess baby at 6 months of age
   E. Assess baby at 12 months of age
2. A baby was born at home and bilateral undescended testis was noted soon after birth, but no action was taken. Both testis were impalpable on the 6-week baby check, and the GP contacts you.
   The most appropriate management is
   A. Assessment by paediatrician within 24 h
   B. Assessment by a paediatric surgeon within 24 h
   C. Assessment by paediatrician within 2 weeks
   D. Assessment by a paediatric surgeon within 2 weeks
   E. Reassessment by GP in 10 weeks
3. A baby was born with unilateral undescended testis.
   At 6 months of age, compared to the contralateral descended testis, the undescended testis is likely to demonstrate increased
   A. Gonocytes
   B. Type A dark spermatogonium
   C. Type A pale spermatogonium
   D. Primary spermatocyte
   E. Round spermatid
4. The parents of a child with unilateral undescended testis are eager to know the risk of undescended testis in relatives.
   The risk is highest in
   A. Maternal half brother
   B. Paternal half brother
   C. Maternal cousin
   D. Paternal cousin
   E. Children of an affected parent
5. During the laparoscopic second stage Fowler-Stephens procedure, you find a resilient looping vas deferens in the ipsilateral inguinal canal
   The most appropriate approach to minimise injury to the vas is
   A. Start with the gubernaculum division
   B. Start developing peritoneal flap with the vas
   C. Mobilise the testis using the vascular pedicle
   D. Sharp dissection to release vas from the canal
   E. Open groin exploration

6.4 Pyloric Stenosis

6. During scrotal exploration, you find a testicular appendix attached to the epididymis.
   In females, the remnant of the embryological origin of this structure causes
   A. Parovarian cyst
   B. Fimbrial cyst
   C. Gartner duct cyst
   D. Bartholin cyst
   E. Nabothian cyst

7. In a 15-year-old boy with unilateral hydrocele, the temperature of the scrotum on the affected side is lower than the abdominal temperature by
   A. 0°
   B. 1°
   C. 3°
   D. 5°
   E. 7°

8. A 15-year-old child with Klinefelter syndrome with gynaecomastia and delayed puberty had a late diagnosis of unilateral undescended testis found to be intraabdominal on laparoscopy.
   The most appropriate next step is
   A. Single-stage open orchidopexy
   B. Single-stage Fowler-Stephens orchiopexy
   C. First stage Fowler-Stephens orchiopexy
   D. First stage Shehata laparoscopic traction orchiopexy
   E. Orchidectomy

6.4 Pyloric Stenosis

1. Ultrasound of a 3-week-old baby with gradually worsening milky vomiting is displayed [Case courtesy of Laughlin Dawes, Radiopaedia.org, rID: 8142]

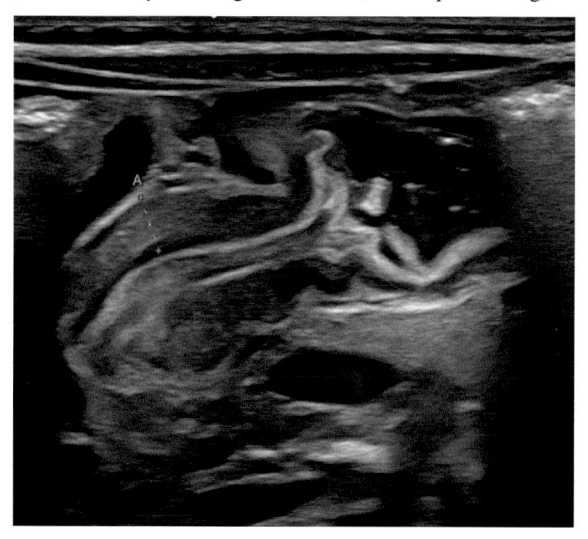

Which sonographic sign is demonstrated
- A. Caterpillar sign
- B. Triangular sign
- C. Stoma sign
- D. Antral nipple sign
- E. Shoulder sign

2. The preoperative ultrasound image is displayed [Case courtesy of Maulik S Patel, Radiopaedia.org, rID: 17284]

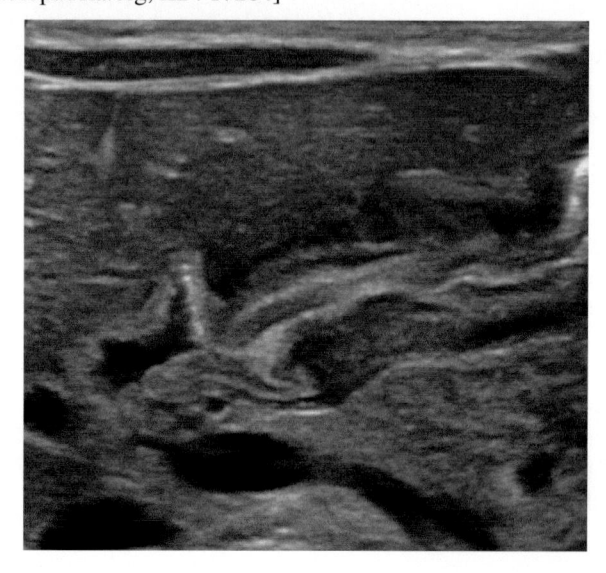

Following surgery, the measurements are likely to return to normal in
- A. 4 weeks
- B. 6 weeks
- C. 12 weeks
- D. 18 weeks
- E. 24 weeks

3. In a baby with pyloric stenosis, surgery is contraindicated due to comorbidities. The medical treatment would constitute
- A. Alpha-adrenergic antagonists
- B. Beta-adrenergic agonists
- C. Beta-adrenergic antagonists
- D. Muscarinic antagoinist
- E. Calcium channel blockers

4. A 2-day-old term neonate with persistent non-bilious vomiting underwent a plain Abdominal X-ray, which only showed a stomach bubble. The skin of the baby easily blisters.
   The best surgical procedure for the baby is:
   A. Billroth 1 operation
   B. Billroth 2 operation
   C. Duodenoduodenostomy
   D. Pyloromyotomy
   E. Gastro jejunostomy

6.5 Bariatric Surgery in Adolescents

1. In the obesity clinic, you would consider bariatric surgery on a 15-year-old with
   A. BMI 31 and Pseudotumor cerebri
   B. BMI 31 with obstructive sleep apnoea
   C. BMI 36 with type 2 diabetes
   D. BMI 36 NASH [non-alcoholic steatohepatitis] activity score [NAS] <3
   E. BMI 39 with no comorbidity
2. A 15-year-old girl with a BMI of 40 and type 2 diabetes has been assessed as a suitable candidate for bariatric surgery.
   The preferred surgery is
   A. Adjustable gastric band (AGB)
   B. Vertical sleeve gastrectomy (VSG)
   C. Roux-en-Y gastric bypass (RYGB)
   D. Biliopancreatic diversion with duodenal switch (BPD/DS)
   E. Primary obesity surgery endoluminal (POSE)
3. While performing a vertical sleeve gastrectomy, you must
   A. Insert a 24 French bougie is inserted along the lesser curvature
   B. Preserve the short gastric vessels
   C. Start dissection 6cm away from the pylorus
   D. Avoid staple line reinforcement
   E. Finish dissection close to gastroesophageal junction
4. 6 weeks after bariatric surgery, the patient develops acute psychosis.
   The treatment is
   A. Dextrose
   B. Vitamin B1
   C. Vitamin B12
   D. Antibiotics
   E. Calcium

6.6 Intestinal Atresia

1. You are performing a laparotomy on a 4-day-old baby with intermittent bilious vomiting whose contrast study is displayed

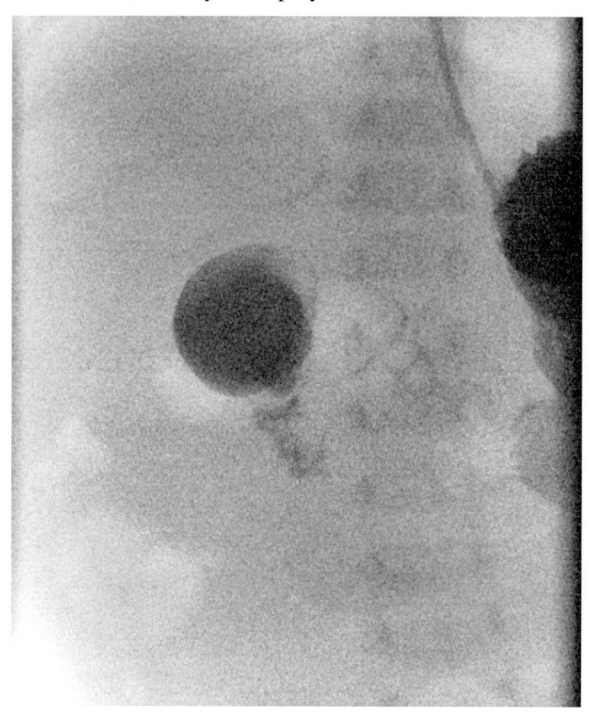

   The correct position of the proximal enterotomy is confirmed by
   A. Visualising bile
   B. Flushing with saline
   C. Passing a feeding tube proximally
   D. Passing a feeding tube distally
   E. Advancing the nasogastric tube through enterotomy

2. During antenatal scanning, the amniotic fluid index was 30 cm
   The most common cause is
   A. Intestinal atresia
   B. Twin pregnancy
   C. Gestational diabetes
   D. Rhesus disease
   E. Infection

3. During endoscopy for upper GI bleeding, a bleeding duodenal ulcer was demonstrated
   The bleeding is likely to be from
   A. Gastroduodenal artery
   B. Supraduodenal artery
   C. Superior pancreaticoduodenal artery
   D. Inferior pancreaticoduodenal artery
   E. Superior mesenteric artery
4. A 14-year-old child had recovered from a complicated appendicitis represented with intermittent bilious vomiting. The contrast study is displayed. NJ Attempt failed and no clinical improvement was observed after 6 weeks of parenteral nutrition.

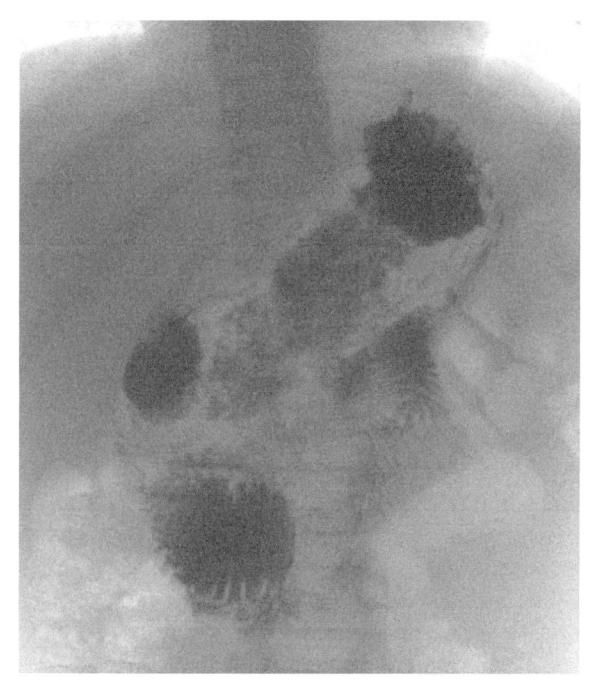

   The next step in management is
   A. Surgical jejunostomy
   B. Duodenojejunostomy
   C. Duodenal mobilisation
   D. Balloon dilatation
   E. Duodenal resection and anastomosis

5. A baby with duodenal atresia was diagnosed to have Down's syndrome
   The most significant prognostic factor is
   A. Prematurity
   B. Oesophageal atresia
   C. Cardiac defects
   D. Small bowel atresia
   E. Hirschsprung's disease
6. In a baby with progressive abdominal distension, isolated colonic atresia with a 1:6 discrepancy was found in the most common location.
   The preferred surgical option is
   A. Colostomy with delayed anastomosis
   B. end-to-end colo-colic anastomosis
   C. end-to-end ileocolic anastomosis
   D. tapering and end-to-end colo-colic anastomosis
   E. Imbrication and end-to-end colo-colic anastomosis
7. During the laparotomy in a baby with intestinal obstruction, a type 3b atresia was found.
   Which branch of the superior mesenteric artery is likely to be present
   A. Ileal branches
   B. Jejunal branches
   C. Ileocolic artery
   D. Right colic artery
   E. Middle colic artery

6.7 Meconium Ileus

1. In a baby with meconium ileus, F508del of the CFTR gene was identified.
   The following is expected in the airway lumen.
   A. Increased transcellular sodium secretion
   B. decreased apical membrane bicarbonate secretion
   C. Increased transcellular water secretion
   D. decreased apical membrane potassium secretion
   E. Increased apical membrane chloride secretion
2. The most common cause of male infertility in cystic fibrosis is
   A. Malnutrition
   B. Hypogonadism
   C. Absent vas
   D. Seminal vesicle atrophy
   E. Erectile dysfunction
3. A foetus was found to have echogenic bowel on 20-week scan
   The most likely post-natal outcome is
   A. Normal baby
   B. Small for date
   C. Premature delivery
   D. Cystic fibrosis
   E. Cytomegalovirus

6.7 Meconium Ileus 63

4. Meconium ileus can be treated with a therapeutic enema
   Gastrograffin (meglumine diatrizoate) is more effective than omnipaque (iohexol) as it is
   A. Hyperosmolar
   B. Surface active
   C. Mucolytic
   D. Lubricant
   E. Detergent
5. A baby has surgery for meconium ileus and is currently NBM
   Creon (pancrelipase) is not started before feeds are established to prevent
   A. Mouth ulcers
   B. Gastritis
   C. Diarrhoea
   D. Cholestasis
   E. Colonic stricture
6. An 8-hour-old term baby develops progressive abdominal distension with a tense, shiny abdomen. A plain x-ray is displayed.

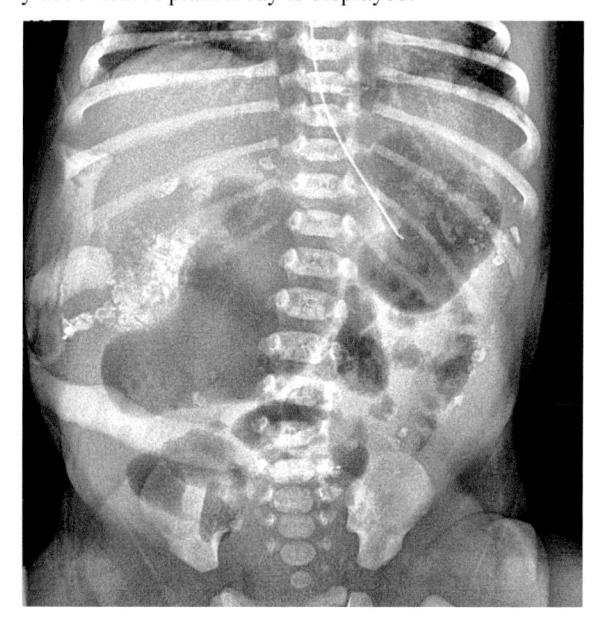

   The next step in the management of the patient is:
   A. Contrast enema
   B. Contrast meal
   C. Rectal washout
   D. Plan for urgent laparotomy
   E. Ultrasound scan

7. A 2-day-old term baby who has failed to pass meconium with progressive abdominal distension is now vomiting bile. He has no features of peritonitis. The next step in the investigation is:
   A. Contrast enema
   B. Contrast swallow
   C. Contrast follow-through
   D. Ultrasound scan
   E. Lateral decubitus film
8. A contrast enema of a 2-day-old baby girl performed for delayed passage of meconium and abdominal distension is displayed. Following the study, the abdominal distension had settled, and the baby had been feeding and opening bowels spontaneously.

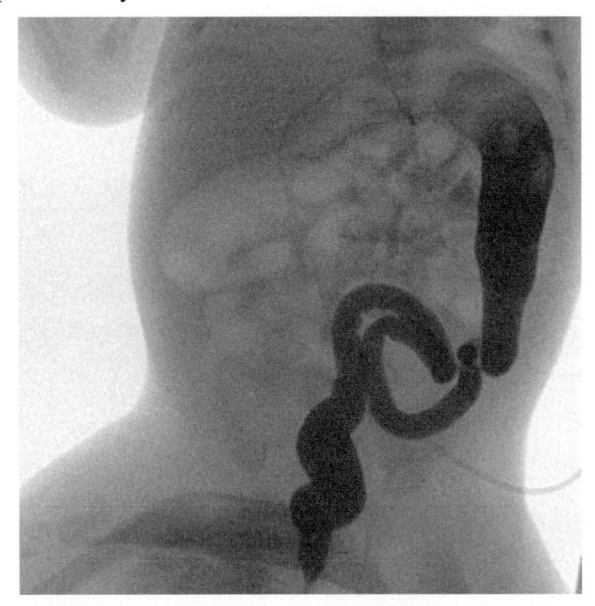

   Which of the following is indicated in the management of this child
   A. N acetylcysteine
   B. Creon
   C. Rectal biopsy
   D. Colostomy
   E. Ileostomy

6.8 Intussusception

1. One-third of the patients have a history of viral illness before the onset of intussusception.
   The most common virus is
   A. Adenovirus
   B. Respiratory syncytial virus
   C. Rotavirus
   D. Enterovirus
   E. Rhinovirus
2. The pathogenesis of intussusception is multifactorial
   Which of the following is protective
   A. Rotavirus infection
   B. Cow's milk based formula
   C. Malnutrition
   D. Previous laparotomy
   E. MMR vaccine
3. Which of the following rotavirus vaccines has the highest risk of intussusception?
   A. Rotarix (derived from a single common strain of human rotavirus)
   B. RotaTeq (a reassorted bovine-human rotavirus)
   C. Rotavac (naturally occurring bovine-human reassortant neonatal G9P, also called 116E)
   D. RotaSiil (bovine-human reassortant with human G1, G2, G3 and G4 bovine UK G6P[5] backbone)
   E. RotaShield (rhesus rotavirus vaccine-tetravalent, RRV-TV)
4. A child with melanocytic macules on the lips, presents with intussusception.
   The most common extraintestinal malignancy associated with this condition is
   A. Breast
   B. Ovarian
   C. Lung
   D. Uterine
   E. Testicular
5. An 8-month-old baby had 45 cm trans-gastric jejunal tube insertion for reflux. The baby started intermittent episodes of screaming and bilious gastric aspirates. Jejunal feeding is tolerated. An upper GI contrast study showed no obstruction.
   The next step in the management is
   A. Fundoplication
   B. Surgical feeding jejunostomy
   C. Shorten trans-gastric jejunal tube
   D. Nasojejunal feeding
   E. Continuous gastrostomy feeds

6. In a 6-year-old child with intussusception, the most common pathological lead point was found.
   The artery that supplies the lead point most commonly originates from
   A. Abdominal aorta
   B. Superior mesenteric artery
   C. Ileal branch of superior mesenteric artery
   D. Ileocolic artery
   E. Internal iliac artery

6.9 Malrotation

1. A 4-day-old term baby attended the emergency department from home with two bilious vomit at 0100 h. Abdominal examination, observations and blood tests are normal. Contrast study is displayed.

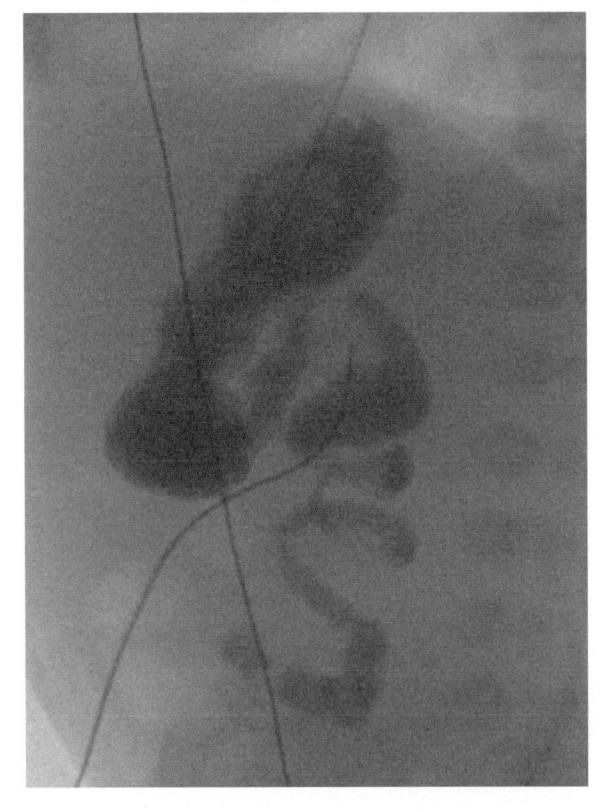

   The most appropriate management is
   A. Delayed AXR
   B. Contrast enema
   C. Immediate Laparotomy
   D. Urgent laparotomy at 0800 h
   E. Panned laparotomy when theatres are available

6.9 Malrotation

2. In a baby with bilious vomiting, an ultrasound scan was performed. Which of the following is most sensitive and specific to rule out malrotation?
   A. SMV right to SMA
   B. SMA right to SMV
   C. SMA anterior to SMV
   D. Demonstration of retro-mesenteric D3
   E. Normal calibre duodenum

3. Most surgeons perform appendicectomy during Ladd's procedure. The reason for appendicectomy is
   A. The appendix has no function
   B. Appendicitis is more common after Ladd's procedure
   C. Appendicosmy ACE procedure not possible in future
   D. Appendicular vessels are likely damaged during the division of Ladd's bands
   E. It prevents intussusception

4. In a 14-year-old child with long-standing abdominal pain, a CT scan was performed which showed internal herniation of small bowel in the right anterior pararenal space behind the ascending colon.

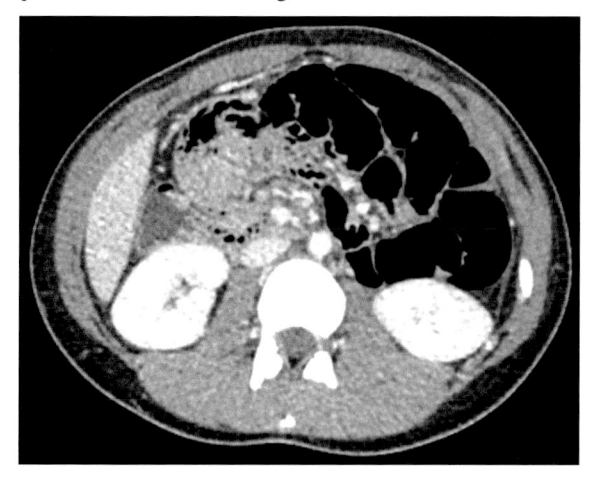

   The treatment is
   A. Ladd's procedure
   B. Reduction of bowel and widening of the neck of the sac
   C. Reduction of bowel and closure of defect
   D. Reduction of the bowel from the sac
   E. Mobilisation of the descending colon

5. A two-day-old term baby presents with green bilious vomiting. On examination, the child is lethargic with a pulse rate of 190/min with rapid shallow breathing. Blood gases: pH 7.1, base excess -8. The child is being resuscitated.
   The next step of action is:
   A. contrast study
   B. Ultrasound
   C. Laparoscopy
   D. Laparotomy
   E. Endoscopy

6. A child is found during laparotomy to have malrotation.
   The primary step of the procedure which prevents recurrent volvulus is:
   A. Widening of the mesentery
   B. Kocherisation of duodenum
   C. Adhesions
   D. Appendicectomy
   E. Dividing the Ladd's bands
7. In a 4-year-old child, during routine screening upper GI contrast study preoperatively for PEG insertion, the stomach capacity and emptying were normal, there was no reflux, and the DJ flexure was found to be at the level of L3.
   The next procedure for the child is:
   A. PEG insertion
   B. Emergency Ladd's procedure
   C. Planned Ladd's procedure
   D. PEG J insertion
   E. Diagnostic Laparoscopy

6.10 Short Bowel Syndrome

1. A child with short bowel syndrome developed renal stones
   The pathophysiology in the bowel lumen leading to this condition is
   A. Decreased bile salt
   B. Increased acidity
   C. Increased fat
   D. Increased free calcium
   E. Increased reducing substances
2. A 5-year-old child on home parenteral nutrition presents with a fever of 39°C, lethargy, metabolic acidosis, hypoglycemia, and thrombocytopenia. Paired quantitative blood cultures were taken simultaneously from both the CVC and a peripheral vein.
   The next step of management is antibiotics of the following type
   A. Glycopeptide
   B. Lincosamides
   C. Macrolides
   D. Nitroimidazoles
   E. Quinolones
3. Gastric hypersecretion in the short bowel is most commonly seen after jejunal resection due to
   A. Decreased VIP
   B. Increased CCK
   C. Increased GIP
   D. Increased secretin
   E. Increased serotonin

4. Cholelithiasis in short-bowel syndrome is more common after resection of
   A. Ileocaecal valve
   B. Mid-jejunum
   C. Proximal ileum
   D. Proximal jejunum
   E. Terminal ileum
5. Small intestinal bacterial overgrowth (SIBO) is more commonly seen in children with short bowel after resection of
   A. Colon
   B. Ileocaecal valve
   C. Mid-jejunum
   D. Proximal ileum
   E. Proximal jejunum

6.11 Gastrointestinal Bleeding

1. A 4-year-old child with a previous Kasai procedure for biliary atresia presents with haematemesis.
   The pharmacological therapy, according to BSPGHAN guidelines, includes
   A. Dopamine agonist
   B. Somatostatin agonist
   C. Somatostatin antagonist
   D. Vasopressin agonist
   E. Vasopressin antagonist
2. In a child with variceal bleeding, the bleeding continues after ongoing medical management, and you are inserting a Sengstaken tube. The child weighs 35 Kg
   The correct technique is
   A. 16 Fr tube inserted nasally in awake child, the gastric balloon inflated with 40 ml saline and 10 ml contrast.
   B. 16 Fr tube inserted orally after endotracheal intubation, the gastric balloon inflated with 10 ml saline and 10 ml contrast.
   C. 16 Fr tube inserted orally after endotracheal intubation, the gastric balloon inflated with 40 ml saline and 10 ml contrast.
   D. 18 Fr tube inserted orally after endotracheal intubation, the gastric balloon inflated with 90 ml saline and 10 ml contrast.
   E. 18 Fr tube inserted orally in awake child, the gastric balloon inflated with 90 ml saline and 10 ml contrast.
3. In a 14-year-old child with recurrent epigastric pain and intermittent haematemesis, peptic ulcer disease was identified. Biopsy confirmed h-pylori, but antibiotic susceptibility is unknown.
   The antibiotic regime, according to ESPGHAN and NASPGHAN guidance, is
   A. Amoxicillin and Clarithromycin standard dose for 14 days
   B. Amoxicillin and Clarithromycin standard dose for 28 days
   C. Amoxicillin and Metronidazole standard dose for 14 days
   D. Amoxicillin and Metronidazole high dose for 14 days
   E. Metronidazole and Clarithromycin standard dose for 14 days

4. A toddler presents with painless rectal bleeding. The blood is altered, and haemoglobin drops. You are organising a radionucleotide scan.
   Which of the following could enhance the image?
   A. Betahistine
   B. Desiglucagon
   C. NSAID
   D. Pentagastrin
   E. Prednisolone
5. A 10-year-old boy presents with intermittent fresh rectal bleeding. Colonoscopic evaluation reveals 6 colonic polyps in the rectum and colon, which are hamartomatous on histology. The largest polyp is 8 mm in diameter. SMAD4 mutation was detected
   The next step in management is
   A. Colonoscopy in first-degree relatives
   B. Cyclooxygenase-2 (COX-2) inhibitors
   C. Excision of all polyps
   D. Screening for cerebral and pulmonary AVMs
   E. Total colectomy
6. A 9-year-old with genotype 45, XO, presents with intermittent lower GI bleeding. The most likely cause of the bleeding is
   A. Coagulopathy
   B. Colitis
   C. Polyp
   D. Ulcer
   E. Vascular malformation
7. An otherwise healthy breastfed newborn infant presents with haematochezia associated with persistent mucus-streaked diarrhoea.
   The next step of management is
   A. Amino acid based formula
   B. Cow's milk free diet for mother
   C. Extremely hydrolysed formula
   D. Partially hydrolysed formula
   E. Soy based formula

6.12 Alimentary Tract Duplications

1. During an upper GI endoscopy in a child presenting with dysphagia and retrosternal pain, a spherical bulge in the posterior wall of the oesophagus suspicious of a duplication cyst was found.
   The next investigation for definitive diagnosis is:
   A. Ultrasound scan of the chest
   B. CT scan of the chest
   C. Chest X ray
   D. MRI of the chest
   E. Nuclear scan

2. A child was diagnosed to have a neurenteric cyst of the oesophagus affecting the spinal cord but with no Oesophago gastric symptoms.
   The next step in the management is:
   A. Conservative management
   B. Spinal operation alone
   C. Thoracic operation alone
   D. 2 stage spinal and thoracic operation
   E. 1 stage spinal and thoracic operation
3. The following procedure is done During the operation of an intra-mural oesophageal duplication cyst.
   A. Excision of mucosa only
   B. Excision of the whole cyst
   C. Excision of mucosa and muscle layer only
   D. Aspiration only
   E. Resection and anastomosis of oesophagus
4. A child was found to have multiple abdominal duplication cysts.
   The following associations then should be sought.
   A. Cerebral anomalies
   B. Spinal anomalies
   C. Genital anomalies
   D. Hepatobiliary anomalies
   E. Ear anomalies
5. A child with a presacral duplication cyst presents with an abscess in the area that is not responding to five days of antibiotics.
   The next step in the management is:
   A. Continue antibiotics for another 5 days
   B. Aspiration
   C. Internal drainage of abscess via rectum
   D. External drainage of abscess
   E. Resection of the cyst

6.13 Polypoid Diseases of the Gastrointestinal Tract

1. A 15 year old boy has been diagnosed with Familial Adenomatous Polyposis syndrome:
   The most appropriate step in the management is:
   A. Regular colonoscopy
   B. Total proctocolectomy
   C. Mucosectomy of the colon
   D. Total colectomy, rectal mucosectomy and ileo anal pouch.
   E. Conservative management of symptoms

2. A 7-year-old boy underwent excision of 2 juvenile polyps because of protrusion. The next step in the management is:
   A. Genetic test for FAP
   B. Elective colonoscopy
   C. Urgent colonoscopy
   D. Upper GI Endoscopy
   E. Ultrasound of the abdomen
3. During routine screening of a family with FAP, a 2 year old asymptomatic boy was found to carry an APC gene.
   The next step in the management is:
   A. Immediate screening programme
   B. Screening programme to start at 8 years
   C. Screening programme to start at 3 years
   D. Ultrasound of the abdomen
   E. Urgent colectomy
4. An 11 year old boy with no family history was diagnosed to have FAP.
   The plan for the rest of the family is:
   A. Faecal calprotectin
   B. Colonoscopy
   C. Genetic testing
   D. Ultrasound
   E. No action necessary
5. A 14-year-old boy was diagnosed with FAP after colonoscopy and biopsy.
   Other tumours to look out for in this boy include:
   A. Medulloblastoma
   B. Hepatocellular carcinoma
   C. Gastric cancer
   D. Liposarcoma
   E. Fibrosarcoma
6. A 12 year old boy with FAP is undergoing upper GI endoscopy as a regular surveillance was found to have a sessile duodenal polyp measuring 1.5 cm.
   The next step is
   A. Diathermy ablation of the polyp
   B. Endoscopic removal
   C. Biopsy of the covering mucosa
   D. Duodenotomy and removal of the polyp
   E. Surveillance endoscopy
7. During routine screening in a 12-year-old boy with Peutz Jeghter syndrome, 8 polyps of 1.5 cm diameter were found in the 7 cm length of mid ileum.
   The treatment is:
   A. Resection of affected bowel
   B. Biopsy of one of them
   C. Removal of most of them
   D. Removal of all of them
   E. Conservative management

8. A 14 year old girl is diagnosed with Peutz Jeghter syndrome.
   The surveillance protocol includes:
   A. Yearly breast and pelvic examinations with cervical smears
   B. Yearly upper and lower GI endoscopy
   C. Biennially Pancreatic ultrasound
   D. Yearly contrast follow through
   E. 6 monthly Full Blood Count

6.14 Necrotising Enterocolitis

1. A preterm neonate is being treated for NEC with optimum medical therapy. 48 h later, CRP is 90, the baby has to be moved to High-Frequency Oscillatory Ventilation and is on Dopamine IV 20 micrograms/kg/min, Dobutamine IV 20 micrograms/kg/min, and Adrenaline IV 100 nanograms/kg/minute The abdominal X-ray demonstrated NEC but no perforation.
   The next step in the management is:
   A. Laparotomy
   B. Continuing medical therapy
   C. Withdrawal of care
   D. Probiotics
   E. Change antibiotics
2. During a laparotomy for NEC, patchy necrosis of the bowel was found. There was 25 cm of viable bowel, 18 cm of doubtful bowel, and the rest was necrotic.
   The next step is:
   A. Excise dead and doubtful bowel
   B. Closure of the abdomen
   C. Excise dead bowel
   D. Primary anastomosis
   E. Excise dead bowel and stoma
3. The parents of a post-operative child recovering from surgery for spontaneous intestinal perforation would like to know links and associations to be careful with for subsequent pregnancies.
   The following is an association.
   A. Steroids
   B. Vitamin A
   C. Smoking
   D. Alcohol
   E. Sodium Picosulphate
4. In the early post-natal period of a premature neonate on steroids for the premature lungs, the following has a protective effect on spontaneous intestinal perforation.
   A. Enteral feeding
   B. Nil by mouth
   C. Indomethacin
   D. Milk fortifiers
   E. Parenteral nutrition

5. There is a significant increase in the abundance of Enterobacteriaceae colonising the gut of NEC infants than those of controls.
   Which of the following is identified as one of the dominating taxon
   A. Klebsiella
   B. Proteus
   C. Salmonella
   D. Serratia
   E. Yersinia
6. The gas in the pneumatosis intestinalis mainly consists of
   A. Nitrogen
   B. Hydrogen
   C. Hydrogen sulphide
   D. Methane
   E. Carbon dioxide
7. Which of the mycobacterial genera present in breastmilk has a protective role in NEC
   A. Gemella
   B. Prevotella
   C. Bifidobacterium
   D. Propionibacterium
   E. Ralstonia
8. A baby with previously medically treated NEC presents with ongoing abdominal distension. A contrast enema was performed.

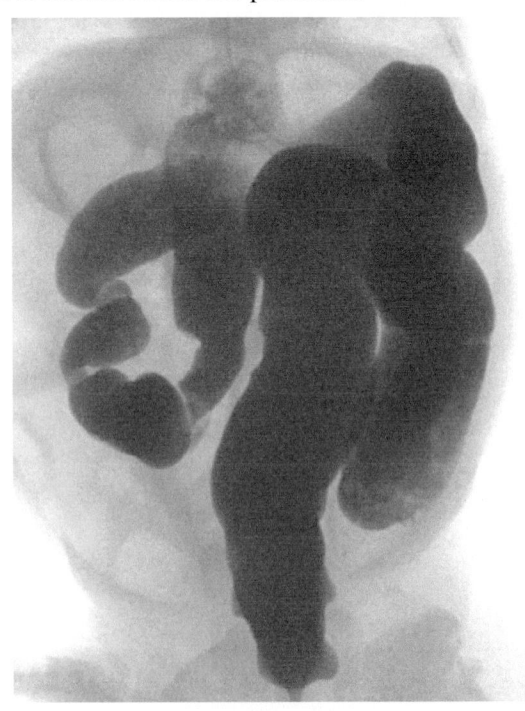

The next step in management is
A. Rectal biopsy
B. Bowel resection
C. Stoma formation
D. Gut decontamination
E. Parenteral nutrition

6.15 Inflammatory Bowel Disease

1. A 14-year-old boy with known ulcerative colitis is admitted with acute severe colitis. The stool culture showed the most commonly identified organism.
   The recommended antibiotic is
   A. Ciprofloxacin
   B. Gentamicin
   C. Metronidazole
   D. Penicillin
   E. Vancomycin

2. The gene associated with paediatric Crohn's disease and involved in the inflammatory reaction to COVID-19 is located in chromosome 16q12.
   The mutation of this gene in Crohn's disease is associated with
   A. Better response to medical treatment
   B. Colonic disease
   C. Ileal disease
   D. No effect on prognosis
   E. Perianal disease

3. The stool concentration of a member of the S100 protein family is used to diagnose inflammatory bowel disease.
   The highest concentration of the protein is found in the cytoplasm of
   A. Basophil
   B. Eosinophil
   C. Erythrocytes
   D. Macrophage
   E. Neutrophil

4. A child with Crohn's disease presents with renal stones.
   The most likely composition of the stone is
   A. Cysteine
   B. Oxalate
   C. Phosphate
   D. Struvite
   E. Urate

5. A 12-year-old child with known Crohn's disease had the following imaging.

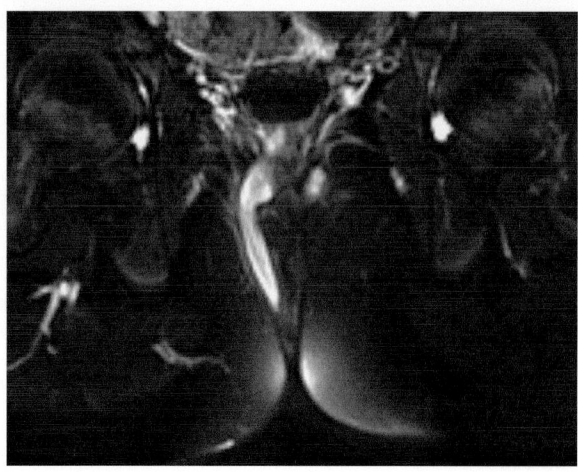

The most. appropriate treatment is
A. Bowel resection
B. Incision and drainage
C. Infliximab
D. Seton
E. Stoma formation

6. A 14-year-old boy with Crohn's disease on infliximab therapy presents with abdominal pain and vomiting. The imaging was obtained.

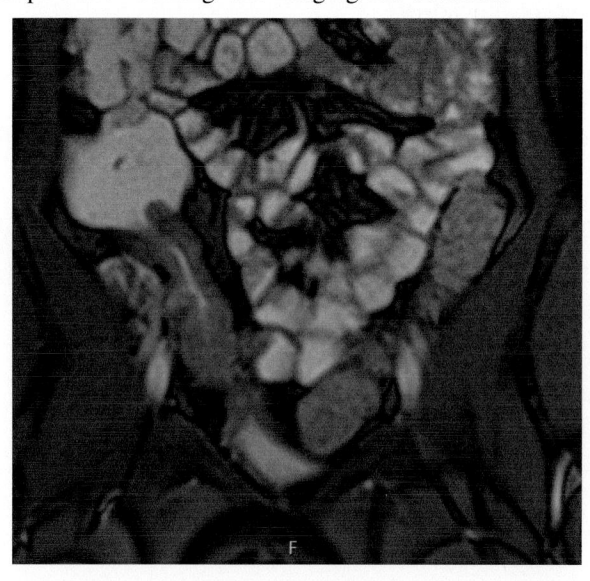

6.15 Inflammatory Bowel Disease

The most appropriate treatment is
A. Methotrexate
B. Radiological drainage
C. Resection
D. Steroids
E. Stoma formation

7. A 10-year-old girl with newly diagnosed Crohn's disease was started on first-line induction therapy.
The anti-inflammatory effect of this treatment is due to
A. Interferon-alpha (IFN-α)
B. Interleukin 10 (IL10)
C. Macrophage inflammatory protein-1 alpha (MIP-1α)
D. Transforming growth factor-beta (TGF-β)
E. Tumor Necrosis Factor Alpha (TNF-α)

8. An 11-year-old girl was newly diagnosed with ulcerative colitis. The Pediatric Ulcerative Colitis Activity Index (PUCAI) score is 25.
The first line of management is
A. 5-ASA
B. Azathioprine
C. Infliximab
D. Prednisolone
E. Vedolizumab

9. A 13-year-old boy with Crohn's disease presents with right iliac fossa pain and pyrexia. A CT scan was obtained.

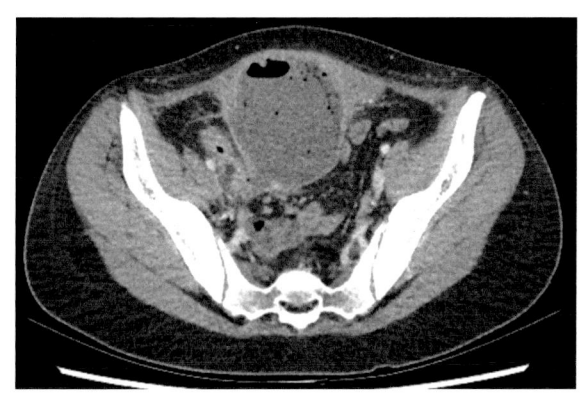

What is the next step in management?
A. Bowel resection
B. Infliximab
C. Laparoscopic washout
D. Percutaneous drainage
E. Stoma formation

10. Chronologically, the first extraintestinal manifestation of inflammatory bowel disease in children is
    A. Aphthous stomatitis
    B. Axial arthropathy
    C. Erythema nodosum
    D. Peripheral arthritis
    E. Uveitis

6.16 Appendicitis

1. You are discussing the treatment of appendicitis with the mother of a 12-year-old girl. She is concerned about future pregnancy.
   The risk of requiring later IVF treatment is increased in
   A. Pelvic appendicitis
   B. Appendicular mass
   C. Appendicular abscess
   D. Medical treatment of appendicitis
   E. No increased risk of requiring IVF
2. A 5-year-old child had a positive cellophane tape test after appendicectomy for uncomplicated appendicitis.
   The treatment is
   A. Praziquantel 5–10 mg/kg single dose
   B. Mebendazole 100 mg single dose
   C. Mebendazole 100 mg twice daily for 3 days
   D. Albendazole 400 mg single dose
   E. Albendazole 400 mg twice daily for 3 days
3. An ultrasound scan of a 12-year-old girl presenting with 24 h of abdominal pain is displayed. The diameter of the structure is 8 mm. She is apyrexial, and her blood tests are normal. However, she has deep tenderness in the right lower quadrant with no guarding.

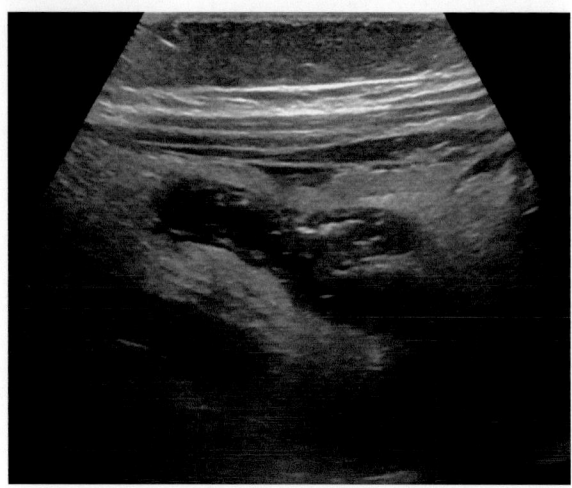

The next step of management is
A. Discharge
B. Observe for 24 h
C. Appendicectomy
D. CT
E. MRI

4. During appendicectomy, you have ligated the appendicular artery. However, during dissection near the base of the appendix, you encounter brisk arterial bleeding.
   The bleeding artery is most likely to originate from
   A. Ileocoloc artery
   B. Anterior caecal artery
   C. Posterior caecal artery
   D. Colic branch of the ileocolic artery
   E. Ileal branch of the ileocolic artery

5. An 8-year-old boy had an appendicectomy for uncomplicated appendicitis. Histology of the appendix demonstrated a 5 mm lesion near the base of the appendix involving the mesoappendix which is synaptophysin positive.
   The next step of management is
   A. Right hemicolectomy
   B. MRI of the abdomen
   C. 24-h urine for 5-hydroxyindoleacetic acid (5-HIAA)
   D. Chromogranin A levels in the blood
   E. No investigations or surgery necessary

6.17 Hirschsprung Disease

1. A newborn diagnosed with Hirschsprung's was found to have a mutation in the PHOX2B gene located on chromosome 4p13
   The baby is most likely to require
   A. Ventriculoperitoneal shunt
   B. Mitrofanoff
   C. Cardiac surgery
   D. Tracheostomy
   E. Deep brain stimulation

2. A 2-year-old child with poliosis has Hirschsprung's disease
   The child is also expected to have
   A. Hydronephrosis
   B. Epilepsy
   C. Deafness
   D. Hydrocephalus
   E. Cardiac septal defects

3. A 3-day-old baby had failed to pass meconium since birth and the abdomen was distended. A contrast study was performed. Partial decompression was achieved after the contrast

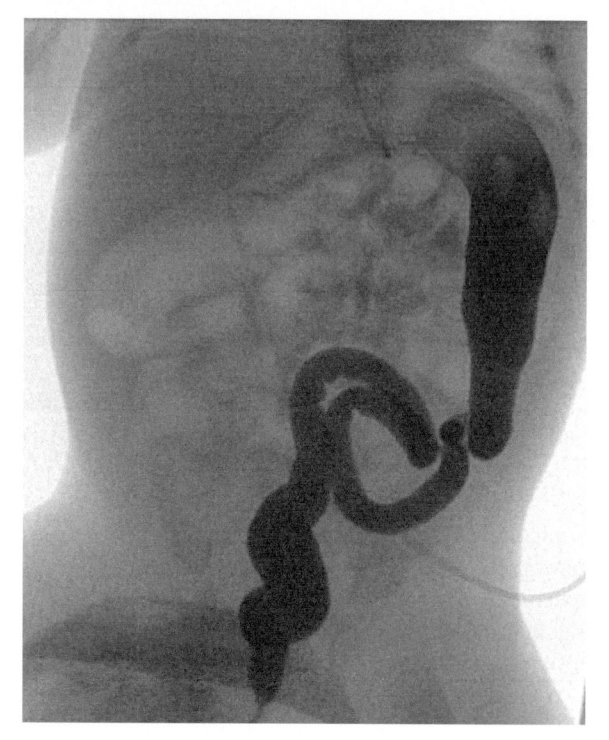

   The next step in management is
   A. Rectal biopsy
   B. Cystic fibrosis genetics
   C. Therapeutic enema
   D. Ileostomy
   E. Transverse colostomy
4. Anorectal manometry was performed on a 5-year-old child with refractory constipation.
   Which of the following findings would suggest Hirschsprung's disease
   A. Negative rectoanal pressure gradient
   B. Decreased squeeze Pressure
   C. Increased basal rhythmic contraction of the anal canal
   D. Absent recto-anal Inhibitory Reflex
   E. High rectal compliance
5. In a rectal biopsy, which is confirmative of hirschsprung's disease?
   A. Acetylcholinesterase increased, Calretinin negative, Peripherin negative
   B. Acetylcholinesterase increased, Calretinin positive, Peripherin positive
   C. Acetylcholinesterase decreased, Calretinin negative, Peripherin positive
   D. Acetylcholinesterase decreased, Calretinin positive, Peripherin negative
   E. Acetylcholinesterase decreased, Calretinin positive, Peripherin positive

6. The contrast enema of a 4-day-old baby girl with Hirschsprung's disease is displayed.

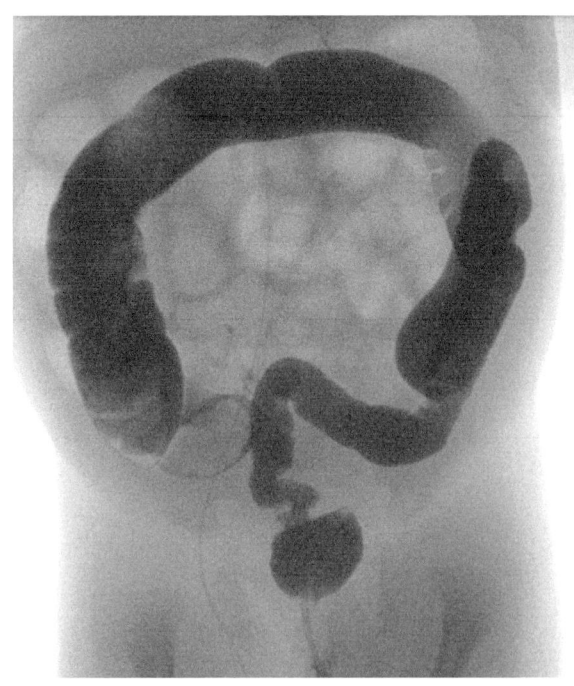

The most appropriate initial surgery is
A. Descending colostomy
B. Transverse colostomy
C. Ileostomy
D. Pull-through
E. Kimura procedure

6.18 Anorectal Malformations

1. A newborn with the 47XY+21 genotype was found to have an anorectal malformation.
   What is the most common type of anomaly
   A. Rectoperineal fistula
   B. Rectourethral fistula
   C. Rectobladderneck fistula
   D. Anorectal atresia with no fistula
   E. Rectal stenosis

2. A baby born with anorectal malformation was found to have a bony abnormality The most commonly affected bone is
   A. Thoracic spine
   B. Lumbar spine
   C. Sacrum
   D. Radius
   E. Ulna
3. A term male neonate was born with an isolated imperforate anus with no other associated anomalies. The x-ray was taken on day 2 of life.

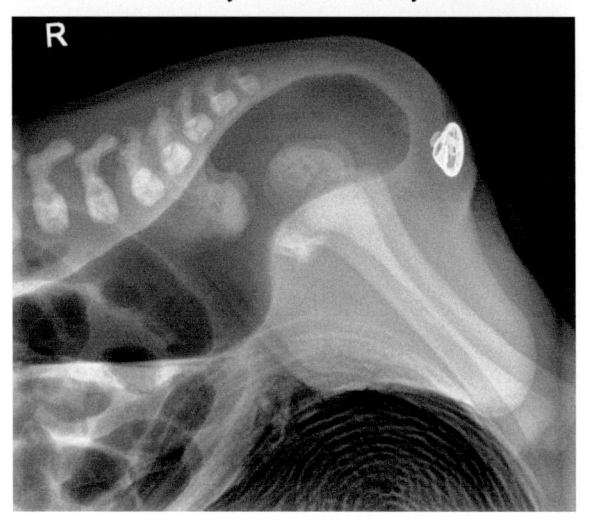

   What is the most appropriate next step in management?
   A. PSARP
   B. Split descending colostomy
   C. Loop descending colostomy
   D. MCUG
   E. Review after 24h

6.18 Anorectal Malformations

4. A baby had a colostomy for anorectal malformation. The following image was performed at six weeks of age

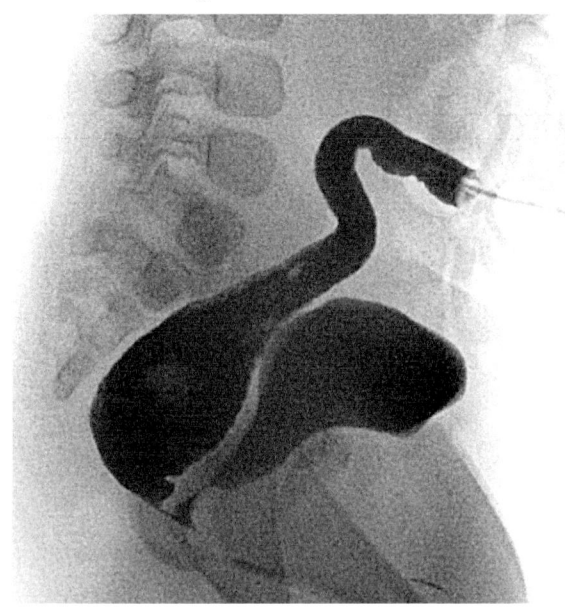

   What is the most appropriate surgical approach?
   A. Perineal only
   B. Perineal followed by abdominal
   C. Abdominal followed by perineal
   D. Simultaneous abdominal and perineal
   E. Abdominal only

5. A baby was born with an anorectal malformation, and subepithelial meconium was noticed in the median raphe of the scrotum.
   What is the most appropriate next step in management?
   A. PSARP
   B. Split descending colostomy
   C. Loop descending colostomy
   D. MCUG
   E. Review after 24h

6. A baby was born with a posterior cloaca with a single perineal opening. The urogenital sinus is approached during repair via
   A. Abdomen
   B. Symphysiotomy
   C. Transperineal anterior to anus
   D. Transrectal
   E. Circumferential mobilisation of anus

7. A female neonate was born with a single perineal opening with hypertrophic folds of skin in the area of a single tiny orifice and a not well-defined anal impression. A suprapubic mass is palpable. The baby had bilateral megaureters on antenatal scans.
   The most appropriate management to prevent urosepsis until definitive surgery is
   A. Split descending colostomy and intermittent urinary catheterisation
   B. Split descending colostomy and indwelling urinary catheter
   C. Split descending colostomy and vesicostomy
   D. Split descending colostomy and ureterostomies
   E. Split descending colostomy, vesicostomy and vaginostomy
8. In a baby with anorectal malformation, the sacral ratio was 0.25.
   The expected final functional prognosis is
   A. Definite constipation
   B. Constipation likely
   C. Definite faecal incontinence
   D. Faecal incontinence likely
   E. Normal bowel function
9. A male infant was born with anorectal malformation. On examination a subepithelial tract filled with meconium that extends into the scrotal raphe was found. The likelihood of this child to be totally continent (voluntary bowel movements and no soiling) in future is
   A. 100%
   B. 80%
   C. 50%
   D. 30%
   E. 10%
10. In a baby with anorectal stenosis, x-ray shows scimitar sacrum.
    The most likely associated lesion is
    A. Teratoma
    B. Meningocele
    C. Hamartoma
    D. Ganglioneuroma
    E. Ependymoma
11. A baby with a recto bladder neck fistula is screened for VACTERL association.
    The most commonly associated anatomic urologic malformation is
    A. Absent kidney
    B. Ectopic Kidney
    C. Hydronephrosis
    D. Hypospadias
    E. Undescended testis

12. An adult male was investigated for ejaculatory dysfunction. He had surgery for a recto bladder neck fistula as a baby.
    The most common cause of the ejaculatory dysfunction is
    A. Ectopic verumontanum
    B. Levator ani syndrome
    C. Psychological
    D. Spinal dysraphism
    E. Urinary sphincter anomaly

6.19 Biliary Atresia and Choledochal Cyst

1. A 4-week-old baby presents with prolonged conjugated jaundice and acholic stools.
   Which is the most accurate investigation to confirm the diagnosis of biliary atresia?
   A. Hepatobiliary Scintigraphy
   B. Endoscopic Retrograde Cholangiopancreatography (ERCP)
   C. Magnetic Resonance Cholangiopancreatography (MRCP)
   D. Liver Biopsy
   E. Peri-Operative Cholangiogram
2. A baby underwent a Kasai portoenterostomy for Biliary Atresia
   Which of the following factors is associated with improved prognosis?
   A. Above 90 days at the initial operation
   B. Syndromic Variety of Biliary Atresia
   C. CMV IgM Positive Associated Biliary Atresia
   D. Cystic Biliary Atresia
   E. Visible Ductal Structures at the Hilum
3. During surgery for biliary atresia in a baby, multiple spleens were identified.
   The other anomaly that may also be encountered is
   A. Annular pancreas
   B. Pre-duodenal portal vein
   C. Duodenal atresia
   D. Left upper lobe agenesis of lungs
   E. Dysplastic kidney

4. The following investigation was performed on an 8 week old baby with conjugated hyperbilirubinemia.

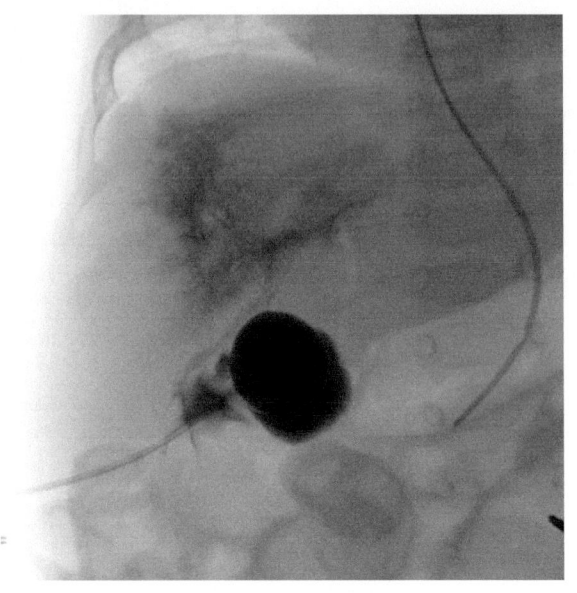

   The next step in the management of this baby is
   A. Liver transplant
   B. Kasai portoenterostomy
   C. Choledochojejunostomy
   D. Choledochoduodenostomy
   E. Hepatic ductoplasty
5. A baby with biliary atresia was found to be IgM Positive for a double-stranded DNA virus associated with poorer prognosis with respect to jaundice clearance. The mechanism of action of the antiviral drug used in this condition is
   A. Inhibition of virus attachment/entry
   B. Inhibition of viral replication
   C. Inhibition of viral protein synthesis
   D. Inhibition of viral assembly
   E. Inhibition of release
6. In a 2-month-old baby with conjugated hyperbilirubinemia, alpha-1 antitrypsin was normal, the TORCH screen was negative, an ultrasound showed a normal gallbladder, and the liver biopsy was equivocal. Therefore diagnostic laparotomy was organised. Clear fluid was aspirated from the gall bladder.
   The next step in management is
   A. Intraoperative cholangiogram
   B. Portoenterostomy
   C. Choledochoduodenostomy
   D. Choledochojejunostomy
   E. ERCP

6.19 Biliary Atresia and Choledochal Cyst 87

7. A 4-year-old boy presents with recurrent abdominal pain. His imaging is shown

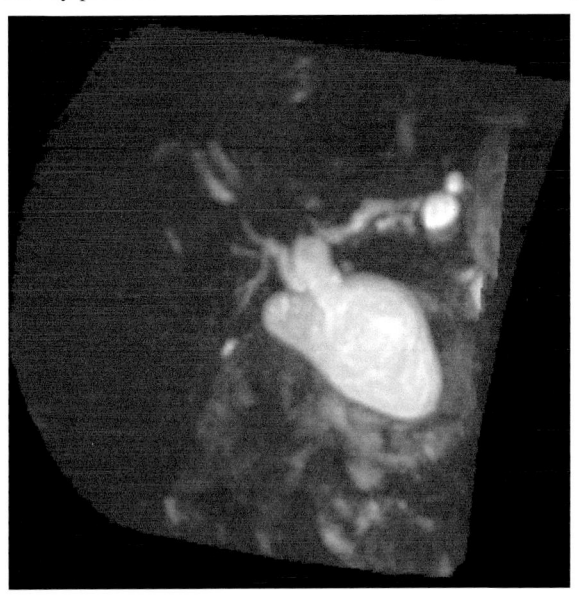

   Which surgery to treat this condition is associated with a higher rate of gastric cancer?
   A. Hepaticojejunostomy
   B. Hepaticoduodenostomy
   C. Choledochojejunostomy
   D. Choledochoduodenostomy
   E. Cyst marsupialisation
8. A 15-year-old girl with autosomal recessive polycystic kidney disease presents with recurrent episodes of fever, jaundice and abdominal pain unresponsive to antibiotics. Her eGFR of 16 ml/min. Her imaging is shown.

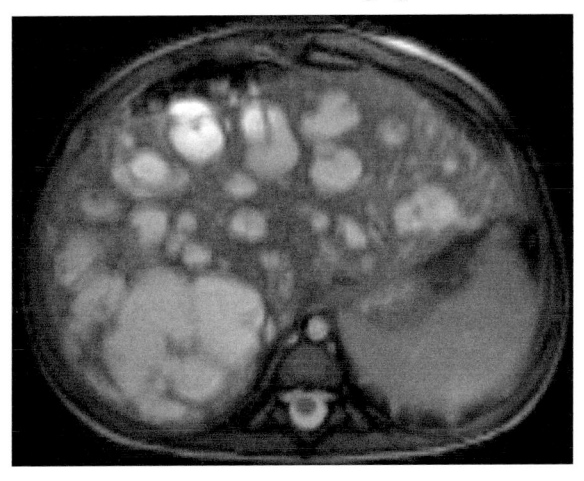

Which is the most appropriate management
A. Internal biliary drainage
B. Hepaticojejunostomy
C. Right Hepatectomy
D. Liver Transplant
E. Combined liver-kidney transplantation

6.20 Gallbladder Disease

1. A 2-year-old child was incidentally diagnosed with gallstones. He was born at 32 weeks of gestation and had type IIIA ileal atresia. He had a prolonged period of nil-by-mouth and parenteral nutrition.
   The most likely composition of the stone is
   A. Cholesterol
   B. Calcium carbonate
   C. Black pigment ($\geq 50\%$ Bilirubin)
   D. Black pigment ($>50\%$ Protein)
   E. Brown pigment

2. A 1-year-old child presents with a high remittent fever, bilateral conjunctivitis, strawberry tongue, cervical lymphadenopathy and generalised rash.
   What is the most common finding of abdominal ultrasound?
   A. Cholecystitis
   B. Gallbladder hydrops
   C. Ascites
   D. Pancreatitis
   E. Hepatitis

3. A child presents with upper abdominal pain, no gallstones were seen on ultrasound, and an abnormal gallbladder ejection fraction (GBEF) on cholecystokinin-stimulated cholescintigraphy.
   The treatment option that is most likely to relieve the symptoms is
   A. Observation
   B. Ursodeoxycholic acid
   C. Corticosteroids
   D. Cholecystectomy
   E. Biliary stent

4. A 10-year-old boy was incidentally diagnosed with an 8 mm pedunculated gallbladder polyp with a thin stalk. He is asymptomatic.
   The most appropriate management is
   A. No follow-up
   B. Ultrasound in 1 month
   C. Ultrasound in 6 months
   D. Ultrasound in 12 months
   E. Cholecystectomy

5. Which cystic duct insertion to the common hepatic duct is associated with the lowest incidence of choledocholithiasis?
   A. Middle-third lateral
   B. Middle-third anterior
   C. Middle-third medial
   D. Proximal-third lateral
   E. Lower-third medial
6. During laparoscopic cholecystectomy, the cystic artery was found to be outside the Calot's triangle
   The most likely origin of the artery is
   A. Right hepatic artery
   B. Aberrant Right hepatic artery
   C. Left hepatic artery
   D. Hepatic artery proper
   E. Gastroduodenal artery
7. A 1-year-old child presents with jaundice, steatorrhoea and pruritus. A liver biopsy suggests progressive familial intrahepatic cholestasis without cirrhosis. The most common initial surgery performed to relieve pruritus is
   A. Partial external biliary diversion
   B. Partial internal biliary drainage
   C. Hepaticojejunostomy
   D. Ileal bypass
   E. Liver transplant
8. In a child presenting with obstructive jaundice and pancreatitis, MRCP demonstrates a CBD stone which could not be extracted by ERCP or laparoscopic CBD exploration.
   What is the next step in the management of the CBD stone?
   A. Percutaneous transhepatic extraction
   B. Hepaticojejunostomy
   C. Whipple procedure
   D. Billroth II gastrectomy
   E. Roux-en-Y gastric bypass
9. Complete transection of CBD was identified intraoperatively during laparoscopic cholecystectomy in an 8-year-old child with hereditary spherocytosis.
   The most appropriate surgical management is management
   A. Direct repair with suturing
   B. Direct repair with suturing over T-tube
   C. Hepaticojejunostomy
   D. Choledochoduodenostomy
   E. Choledochojejunostomy

10. During hepatobiliary iminodiacetic acid (HIDA) scan with intravenous Sincalide, the tracer appears in the extrahepatic bile ducts, but does not enter the cystic duct or the gallbladder
    This finding is suggestive of
    A. Acute Cholecystitis
    B. Chronic Cholecystitis
    C. Biliary dyskinesia
    D. Biliary atresia
    E. Obstructed bile duct

6.21 Portal Hypertension

1. A 4-year-old male child presents with oesophageal variceal bleeding and splenomegaly. He was born prematurely at 32 weeks of gestation and had an umbilical venous catheter.
   Which of the following could have contributed to this
   A. Umbilical catheter tip in the right atrium
   B. Umbilical catheter tip on T8 vertebral body
   C. Umbilical Catheter in situ for one week
   D. Blood transfusion through the umbilical catheter
   E. Parenteral nutrition through the umbilical catheter
2. A fifteen-year-old girl on oral contraceptive pills develops acute abdominal distension and right upper quadrant pain. Ultrasound demonstrates ascites and hepatomegaly with heterogenous liver and no flow in the right hepatic vein. Anticoagulation, thrombolysis and stenting have failed to resolve the symptoms.
   The next line of treatment is
   A. Liver transplant
   B. Proximal Splenorenal Shunt
   C. End-to-side portacaval shunt
   D. Side-to-Side Portacaval Shunt
   E. extracorporeal liver resection, and autotransplantation
3. A 2-year-old child who previously had Kasai porto-enterostomy presents with one episode of haematemesis. The child already had an NG tube and was started on octreotide infusion after fluid resuscitation. No further bleeding was observed on NG aspirates.
   Your next step in managing the child is
   A. Endoscopy
   B. Observation
   C. Spironolactone
   D. Prophylactic Sengstaken tube
   E. TIPS

6.21 Portal Hypertension

4. A seven-year-old girl with biliary atresia with a splenic malformation (BASM) has a stable liver disease following a successful Kasai procedure as a baby. However, she developed breathlessness after normal daily activities. Technetium-99m-labelled macro aggregated albumin ((99m)Tc-MAA) scintigraphy showed intrapulmonary shunting.
   The treatment for this condition is
   A. Lung Transplant
   B. Liver Transplant
   C. Portosystemic shunt
   D. Pulmonary arterial coil embolisation
   E. The condition is fatal

5. A four-year-old child with portal hypertension secondary to extrahepatic portal vein thrombosis presents with recurrent upper GI bleeding and frequent mucosal bleeding associated with low platelets.
   The most appropriate treatment is
   A. Splenectomy
   B. Liver transplant
   C. Rex shunt
   D. Bone marrow transplant
   E. CFU-GM

6. An eight-year-old child presents with severe rectal bleeding, On ultrasound scan, inferior vena cava was dilated and portal vein was not identified. A superior mesenteric venogram identified Abernethy type I portacaval shunt.

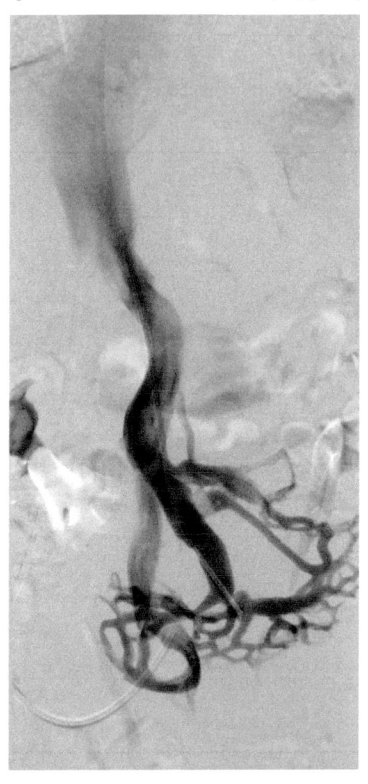

The treatment of this condition is
A. Radiological occlusion
B. Surgical disconnection
C. Liver transplant
D. Meso-Rex shunt
E. Splenectomy

7. A 12-year-old child with ulcerative colitis presents with jaundice and pruritus. MRCP showed a part of CBD to be 1.4 mm in diameter.
   The next line of management is
   A. Prednisolone
   B. Stenting
   C. Choledochoduodenostomy
   D. Choledochojejunostomy
   E. Liver transplant

8. A 7-year-old child with known portal hypertension presents to the emergency department with uncontrolled upper GI bleeding, and you decide to insert a Sengstaken tube.
   Which is the correct procedure?
   A. Insert a 14Fr tube immediately in ED, inflate the gastric balloon with 40mls saline and 10mls contrast, confirm the position of the balloon radiologically, and apply traction to the tube
   B. Intubate the child, insert a 16Fr tube, inflate the gastric balloon with 20mls saline and 20mls contrast, confirm the position of the balloon radiologically, and apply traction to the tube
   C. Intubate the child, insert a 14Fr tube, inflate the gastric balloon with 40mls saline and 10mls contrast, confirm the position of the balloon radiologically, and apply traction to the tube
   D. Intubate the child, insert a 16Fr tube, inflate the gastric balloon and oesophageal balloon with 20mls saline and 20mls contrast, confirm the position of the balloons radiologically, and apply traction to the tube
   E. Intubate the child, insert a 16Fr tube, inflate the oesophageal balloon with 40mls saline and 10mls contrast, confirm the position of the balloon radiologically, and apply traction to the tube

9. A child with no previous upper GI bleeding has a surveillance endoscopy for portal hypertension. Two oesophageal varices are found that would not collapse on inflation of the oesophagus with air, and each would occlude < 1/3 of the oesophageal lumen. There are no stigmata.
   The most appropriate management for the child is
   A. No therapy; repeat endoscopy after 12 months
   B. No therapy; repeat endoscopy after 3–6 months
   C. No therapy; repeat endoscopy after 1–3 months
   D. Band ligation; repeat endoscopy after 1–3 months
   E. Band ligation; repeat endoscopy after 3–6 months

10. During endoscopy for upper GI bleeding, bleeding gastric varices were found. The most appropriate treatment is
    A. Balloon occluded retrograde transvenous obliteration (BRTO)
    B. Banding
    C. Histoacryl glue injection
    D. Sodium tetradecyl sulfate injection
    E. Transjugular intrahepatic portosystemic shunt (TIPS)

6.22 Pancreas

1. A baby was born with the most common congenital anomaly of the pancreas What is the least likely condition the baby may present with in future
    A. Duodenal obstruction
    B. Bilious vomiting
    C. Asymptomatic
    D. Feeding intolerance
    E. Pancreatitis
2. A 2-year-old boy presents with chronic diarrhoea, failure to thrive, and recurrent ear infections. A complete blood count shows anaemia and neutropenia. Secretin-cholecystokinin quantitative stimulation test demonstrates reduced bicarbonate and trypsin production
    Treatment for this condition is
    A. Prednisolone
    B. Water-soluble vitamins
    C. CCK analogue
    D. Pancrelipase
    E. Immunotherapy
3. A 6-year-old boy presents with recurrent pancreatitis, and the MRCP is performed

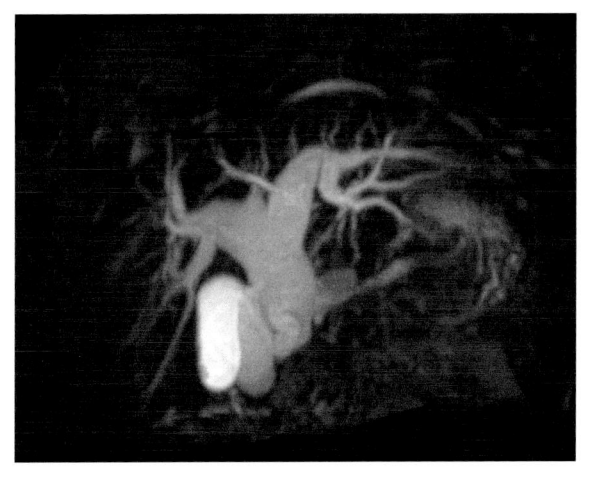

The most appropriate treatment is
   A. Endoscopic papillary balloon dilation
   B. Biliary endoscopic sphincterotomy
   C. Endoscopic bile duct stent
   D. Portoenterostomy
   E. Surgical ampullectomy
4. A 12-year-old girl with hereditary pancreatitis had frequent hospitalisation due to pain despite endoscopic therapy. CT scan show features of chronic diffuse pancreatitis with a dilated pancreatic duct.
   The most appropriate surgical management of the child is
   A. Distal pancreatectomy
   B. Puestow procedure
   C. Whipple Procedure
   D. Beger's procedure
   E. Total Pancreatectomy
5. A newborn baby was admitted to the NICU with irritability, jitteriness and lethargy. The initial blood sugar was unrecordable. Following several glucose boluses, the patient required a dextrose infusion with a GIR (glucose infusion rate) of 16.4mg/kg/min to maintain normal blood sugar. Blood test shows insulin 23.6pmol/L, C peptide 2.2 ng/mL, growth hormone 11.8mcgs/L, cortisol 228nmol/L. The baby was started on Maxijule, Diazoxide, Chlorthiazide and Octreotide, but the high glucose infusion requirement continues.
   Which is the subsequent investigation?
   A. Genetic mutation analysis
   B. PET CT with F-DOPA
   C. MRI of abdomen
   D. Secretin-stimulated magnetic resonance cholangiopancreatography
   E. Optical coherence tomography
6. In a baby with congenital hyperinsulinism not responding to medical treatment, PET CT shows a focal lesion at the head of the pancreas.
   What is the initial step during surgery
   A. Biopsy of the pancreatic tail
   B. Palpation of the lesion
   C. Biopsy of the lesion
   D. Mobilisation of splenic vessels
   E. Mobilisation of duodenum

6.22 Pancreas

7. A 12-year-old boy presents two weeks after a handlebar injury to the abdomen due to increased abdominal pain and vomiting, an MRI is obtained.

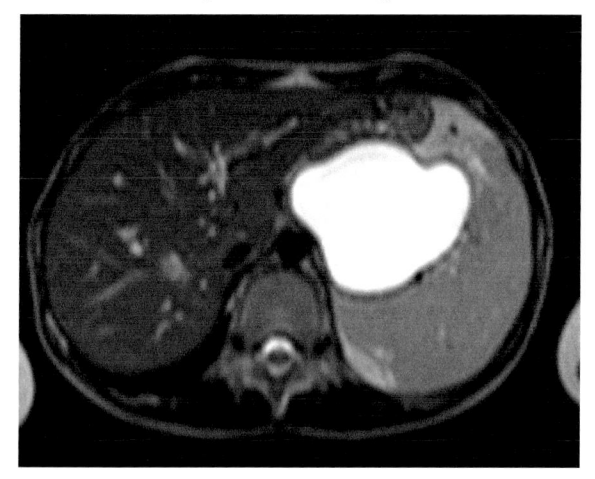

   What is the appropriate initial management?
   A. Endoscopic Cystgastrostomy
   B. Ultrasound-guided drainage
   C. Jejunal feeding
   D. Cystoduodenostomy
   E. Partial pancreatectomy

8. A 4-year-old child presents with chronic voluminous watery diarrhoea, weight loss, and hypokalemia. PET CT demonstrates a pancreatic mass and a normal liver.
   The treatment of choice is
   A. Octreotide
   B. Prednisolone
   C. Streptozocin
   D. Radiofrequency ablation
   E. Resection

9. A 10-year-old child presents with diplopia, blurred vision, palpitations and weakness after fasting or exercising, which improves after taking food. A small solid nodular mass is detected at the tail of the pancreas on helical CT.
   The most common drug used to treat this condition has a common side effect that leads to weight gain. Which drug is used to reduce the side effect?
   A. Glucagon
   B. Hydrochlorothiazide
   C. Prednisolone
   D. Octreotide
   E. Lactulose

10. The most commonly used antiepileptic drug in the UK is one of the most frequent causes of drug-induced pancreatitis. The drug affects an inhibitory neurotransmitter which has role in pain perception.
    The neurotransmitter is
    A. Acetylcholine
    B. Dopamine
    C. Glutamate
    D. Serotonin
    E. Gamma-Aminobutyric acid

6.23 Spleen

1. A child with a history of previous blunt abdominal trauma presents with acute appendicitis. During laparoscopy, multiple small splenic tissues appear to be implanted on the omentum.
   What will be your next step in the management of the omental lesions?
   A. Observation
   B. Biopsy
   C. Omentectomy
   D. Chemotherapy
   E. Radiofrequency ablation

6.23 Spleen

2. A 15-year-old girl presents with acute lower abdominal pain with no peritonitis. She has had several episodes of intermittent, less severe abdominal pain. A CT scan is obtained.

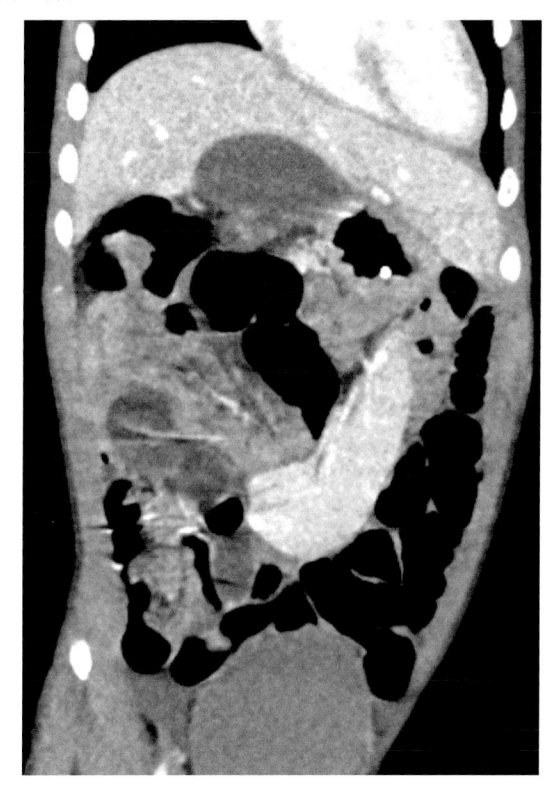

What is the most appropriate management?
A. Observation
B. Splenopexy
C. Splenectomy
D. Oophorectomy
E. Ovarian sparing cystectomy

3. A baby was born with congenital cyanotic heart disease and asplenia. Most likely, the initial cardiac surgical procedure for the baby is
A. Fontan Procedure
B. Glen Procedure
C. Hemi-Fontan Procedure
D. Norwood procedure
E. Heart Transplant

4. During laparoscopy for left impalpable testis, a fibrotic cord with islets of splenic tissue was found connecting the superior pole of the spleen to the superior pole of the intraabdominal testis.
   What is the least likely associated abnormality
   A. Abnormality of femur morphology
   B. Micrognathia
   C. Anal atresia
   D. Congenital diaphragmatic hernia
   E. Oesophageal atresia
5. On ultrasound, an 8-year-old child who recently arrived in the UK from rural South America was incidentally diagnosed with a 3cm multilocular splenic cyst. Blood tests show Eosinophilia and hypogammaglobinemia. ELISA is positive for a parasite.
   The treatment option is not beneficial
   A. PAIR (Puncture, Aspiration, Injection, Re-aspiration)
   B. Surgery
   C. Albendazole
   D. Watch and wait
   E. Pentamidine
6. A 15-year-old is having vaccinations prior to splenectomy for hereditary spherocytosis.
   Which additional vaccine is not administered
   A. PCV13 vaccine
   B. PPV23 vaccine
   C. MenB vaccine
   D. MenACWY conjugate vaccine
   E. Annual influenza vaccine
7. Children with hyposplenism are at risk of overwhelming post-splenectomy infection (OPSI)
   Which is the correct strategy for prophylactic antibiotics
   A. Oral Phenoxymethylpenicillin three times a day
   B. Lifelong antibiotic prophylaxis is not recommended
   C. Antibiotic prophylaxis for a minimum of four years after surgery
   D. Antibiotic prophylaxis up to the age of 10
   E. It can be discontinued after five years in children with sickle cell disease
8. A 2-year-old child with sickle cell disease presents with abrupt onset of pallor, weakness, and tachycardia. Examination reveals a dramatic splenic enlargement beyond their baseline splenomegaly. A blood test shows a rapid drop in the hematocrit with thrombocytopenia.
   The most appropriate strategy to prevent the recurrence of this event is
   A. Prophylactic antibiotics
   B. Prophylactic transfusion
   C. Partial splenectomy
   D. Total splenectomy
   E. Etilefrine

9. Haemolytic anaemias are the most common reason for planned splenectomies in children in the United Kingdom
   According to the British Society of Haematology guidance, which is the correct approach
   A. Laparoscopic and open approaches are equally preferred
   B. Total splenectomy is preferred over partial splenectomy
   C. In children undergoing splenectomy, the gall bladder with incidental gallstones should be removed concomitantly
   D. In children who require cholecystectomy for gallstone symptoms, the use of concurrent splenectomy is controversial
   E. Splenectomy should be done before the age of 10 years
10. A 5-year-old child recently developed easy skin bruises and petechiae. She is otherwise healthy and has no lymphadenopathy or organomegaly. However, the blood count reveals a platelet count of 30×10^9/L with normal haemoglobin, white blood count, and peripheral smear.
    The most appropriate management of the child is
    A. Observation
    B. Prednisone
    C. anti-D immunoglobulin
    D. Rituximab
    E. Splenectomy

Urology

Anindya Niyogi and Alok Godse

7.1 Renal Agenesis, Dysplasia, and Cystic Disease

1. A male fetus is diagnosed with a cystic right kidney. The postnatal ultrasound is displayed

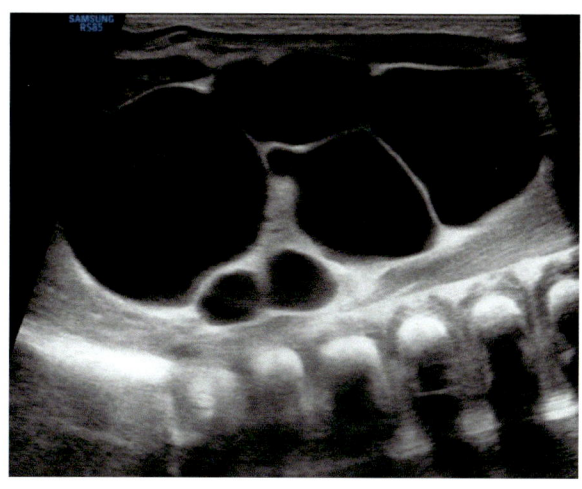

This is likely to be caused by anomalous
 A. Metanephric blastema
 B. Metanephric diverticulum
 C. Mesonephros
 D. Pronephros
 E. Paramesonephric duct

2. In A 2-year-old boy with UTI, a multi-cystic dysplastic left kidney was demonstrated on Ultrasound. No antenatal imaging was available.
 The pathophysiology of this UTI is
 A. PUJO
 B. VUJO
 C. VUR
 D. Ectopic Ureter
 E. Underactive bladder

3. In a 4-year-old girl with intermittent abdominal pain, a horseshoe kidney with bilateral hydronephrosis was detected on ultrasound. MAG3 renogram demonstrated bilateral obstructed curves.
 The most common surgery in this situation is
 A. Retroperitoneal bilateral vascular hitch
 B. Transperitoneal bilateral vascular hitch
 C. Retroperitoneal bilateral dismembered pyeloplasty
 D. Transperitoneal bilateral dismembered pyeloplasty
 E. Transperitoneal bilateral pyeloplasty with renal symphysiotomy

4. MRI of a baby with abdominal distension is displayed.

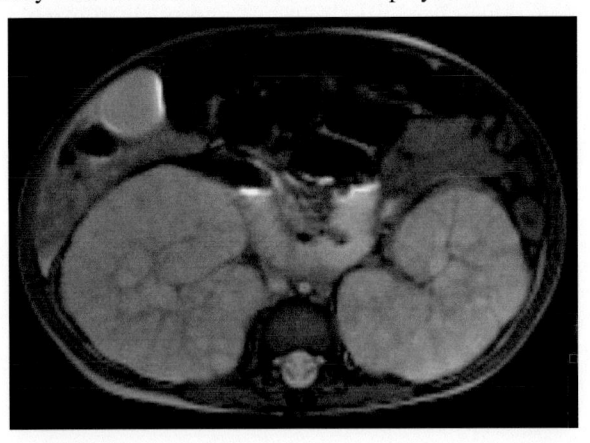

 The most common cause of death in this condition is
 A. Sepsis
 B. Respiratory failure
 C. Cardiac failure
 D. Renal failure
 E. Liver failure

7.1 Renal Agenesis, Dysplasia, and Cystic Disease   103

5. A 6-year-old child with polycystic kidney disease develops hypertension
   The first line of management is
   A. Amlodipine
   B. Atenolol
   C. Chlorothiazide
   D. Doxazosin
   E. Ramipril
6. A fetus is found to have bilateral renal agenesis.
   The risk of a stillborn is:
   A. <10%
   B. 40%
   C. 60%
   D. >90%
   E. 100%
7. A 10-year-old boy presents with abdominal swelling. A CT scan is obtained

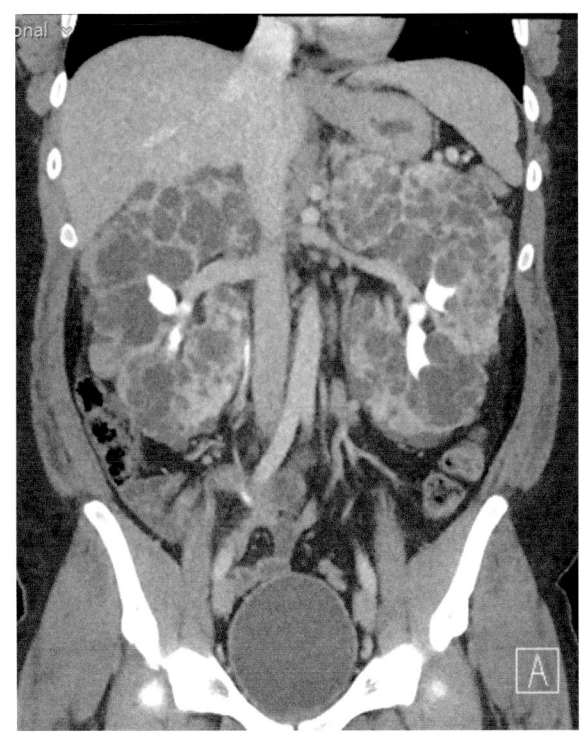

   The most common associated central nervous system anomaly is
   A. Aneurysm
   B. Cysts
   C. Microbleeds
   D. Thrombus
   E. Ventriculomegaly

8. An antenatal scan of a fetus of both parents being carriers for autosomal recessive renal disease is being performed.
   The ultrasound features suggestive of the autosomal recessive polycystic kidney are:
   A. Bilateral dysplastic kidneys
   B. Enlarged hyperechoic kidneys
   C. Enlarged hypoechoic kidneys
   D. Small hyperechoic kidneys
   E. Small hypoechoic kidneys
9. A baby is diagnosed with autosomal recessive polycystic kidney disease. The most common early liver manifestation of the condition is
   A. Caroli disease
   B. Cholangitis
   C. Duct dilatation
   D. Fibrosis
   E. Tumour

7.2 Renal Fusions and Ectopia

10. On an Ultrasound scan of a 5-year-old girl with UTI, a single large right-sided kidney with no hydroureteronephrosis was detected. DMSA images are displayed.

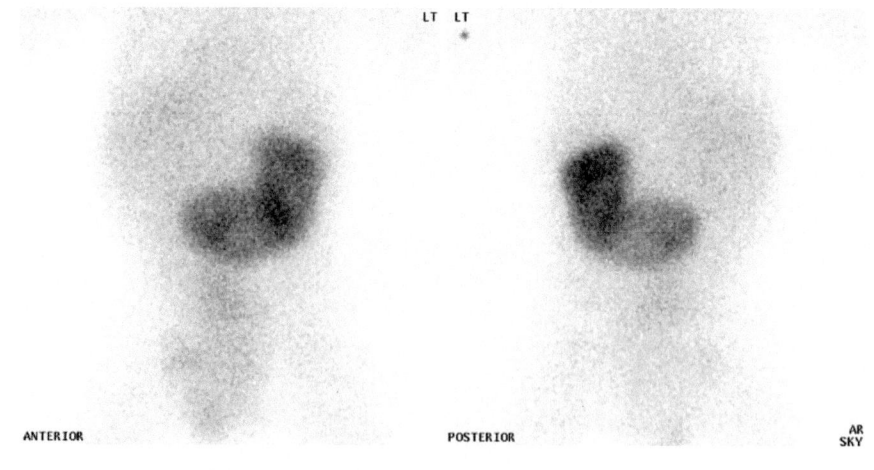

    The most common urological anomaly associated with this condition is
    A. Vesicoureteric reflux
    B. Pelviureteric junction obstruction
    C. Vesicoureteric junction obstruction
    D. Ureteric stricture
    E. Renal dysplasia

7.2 Renal Fusions and Ectopia

11. DMSA scan is displayed

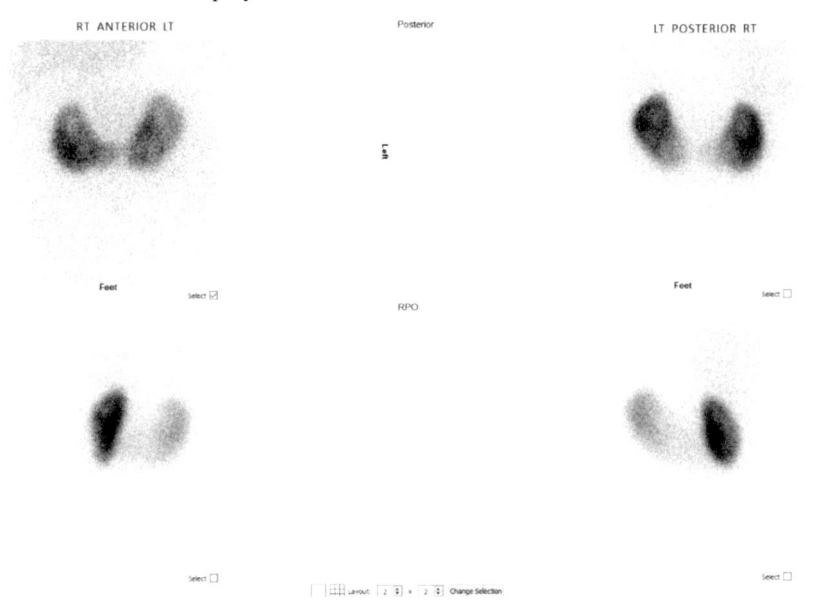

    This anomaly is more common in
    A. 45, XO
    B. 46, XX/XY
    C. 47, XXX
    D. 47, XXY
    E. 47, XYY

12. A 15-year-old male presents with haematuria, and a non-contrast CT scan showed a 10 mm stone within a horseshoe kidney
    The most appropriate treatment is
    A. Laparoscopic approach
    B. Open approach
    C. Percutaneous nephrolithotomy
    D. Shockwave lithotripsy
    E. Ureteroscopic approach

13. In horseshoe kidney, the blood supply to the isthmus is from
    A. Aorta
    B. Common iliac artery
    C. Inferior mesenteric artery
    D. Internal iliac artery
    E. Renal artery

7.3 Pelviureteric Junction Obstruction

1. Renal ultrasound of a newborn baby demonstrated Pelvis: Outside Hilum, Major Calyces: Dilated, Minor Calyces: Uniformly Dilated, Parenchyma: Intact According to the Society for Fetal Urology (SFU), the grade of hydronephrosis is
   A. 1
   B. 2
   C. 3
   D. 4
   E. 5
2. A 2-day-old term baby boy with antenatal right hydronephrosis had an ultrasound scan done on day 2 of life, which demonstrated SFU grade 3 hydronephrosis on the right with no hydroureter and a normal left kidney and bladder. The most appropriate investigation is
   A. Diuretic MAG 3 scan at 8 weeks of life
   B. Diuretic MAG 3 scan within first 2 weeks of life
   C. DMSA scan at 8 weeks of life
   D. DMSA scan within the first 2 weeks of life
   E. Micturating cystourethrogram
3. A fetus was diagnosed with bilateral hydronephrosis on the 20-week anomaly scan The most common cause is
   A. Ectopic ureter
   B. PUJ obstruction
   C. PUV
   D. Transient hydronephrosis
   E. VUR

7.3 Pelviureteric Junction Obstruction

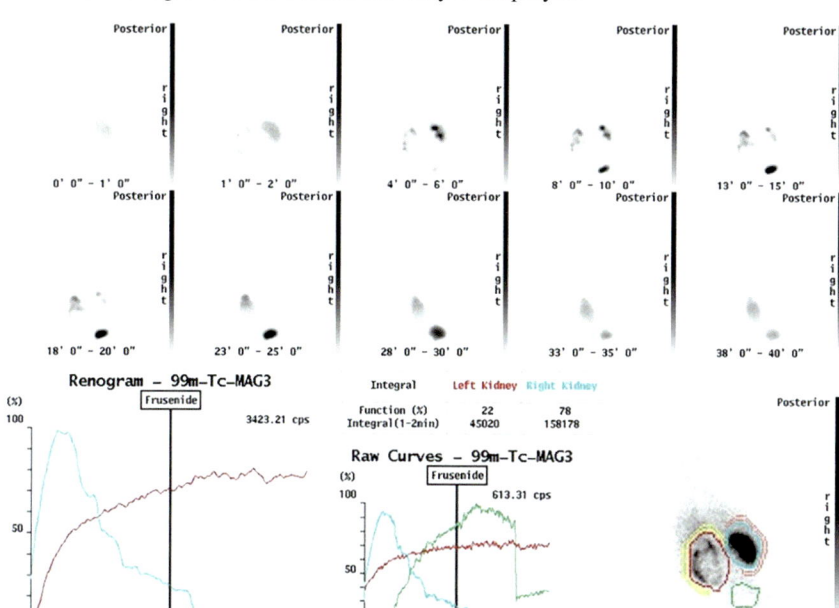

4. MAG3 renogram of a 2-month-old baby is displayed

   The most common aetiology is
   A. Abnormal peristalsis
   B. Crossing lower-pole renal vessel
   C. High insertion of the ureter
   D. Rotation of the kidney
   E. Fibrosis

5. A 7-year-old girl underwent a Laparoscopic left Pyeloplasty 2 weeks ago. A double J stent was inserted at surgery. She is continuously dribbling urine for the last 3 days. She is systemically well and has also been passing urine normally. The best plan of action is
   A. AXR
   B. Nephrostomy
   C. Stent removal
   D. Urethral catheterisation
   E. US KUB

6. Mercaptoacetyltriglycine renogram is preferentially used to assess renal drainage in children because of
   A. 10% protein binding
   B. 70% glomerular filtration
   C. 85% renal distribution
   D. 90% first-pass filtration
   E. 97% tubular secretion

7. MAG3 renogram drainage curve is displayed

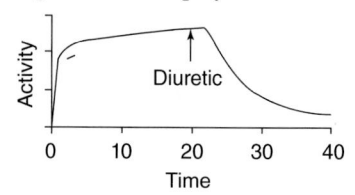

This pattern suggests
A. Delayed decompensation
B. Equivocal
C. Hypotonic pelvis
D. Normal drainage
E. Obstructed drainage

7.4 Vesicoureteral Reflux

1. In a 13-year-old girl with recurrent UTIs and bilateral vesicoureteric reflux, the radionucleotide scan was performed

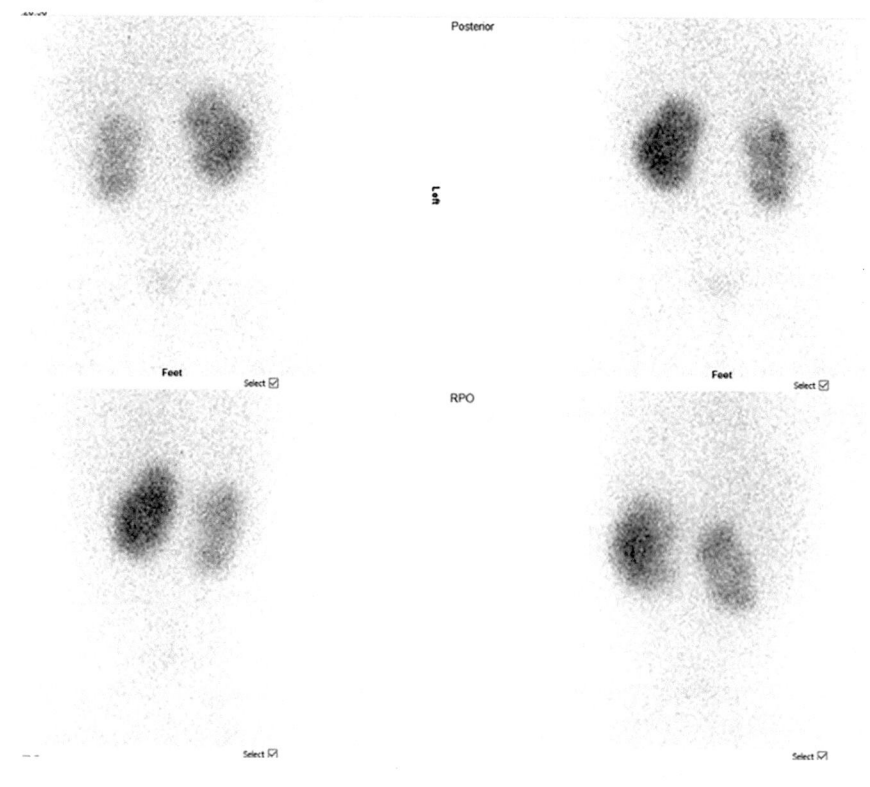

7.4 Vesicoureteral Reflux

The tracer used in the study has the following characteristics.
A. Binds to proximal tubules
B. Secreted by distal tubules
C. Mostly excreted unchanged in urine
D. Low plasma protein binding
E. No glomerular filtration

2. Vesicoureteric reflux is mainly caused by
   A. abnormal bladder function
   B. abnormal trigonal anatomy
   C. ectopic ureteral orifices
   D. bladder outlet obstruction
   E. short intramural ureter

3. A 3-year-old male presents with recurrent breakthrough UTIs. He has no neurological impairment. His MCUG is displayed. There is a significant retention of contrast in both collecting systems after voiding. His DMSA showed bilateral scarring.

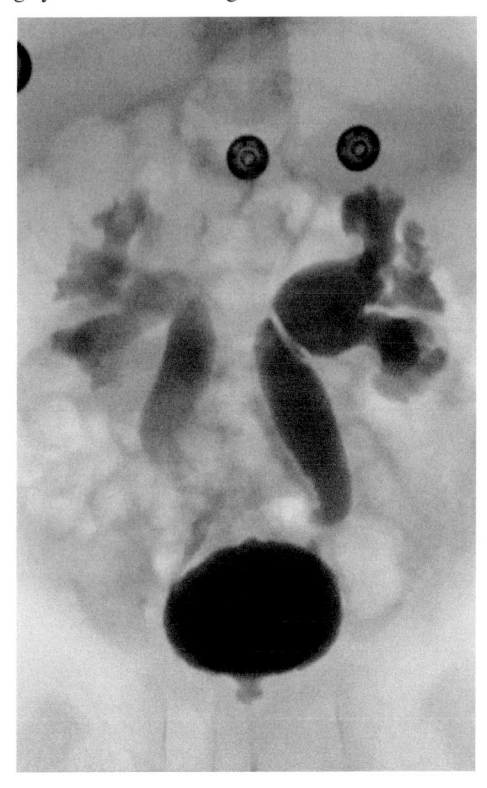

Which is the most appropriate management
A. Cross trigonal reimplantation
B. Hydrodistention Implantation Technique
C. Intermittent catheterisation
D. Loop ureterostomy
E. Vesicostomy

4. A 4-year-old girl with recurrent UTIs had the following investigation

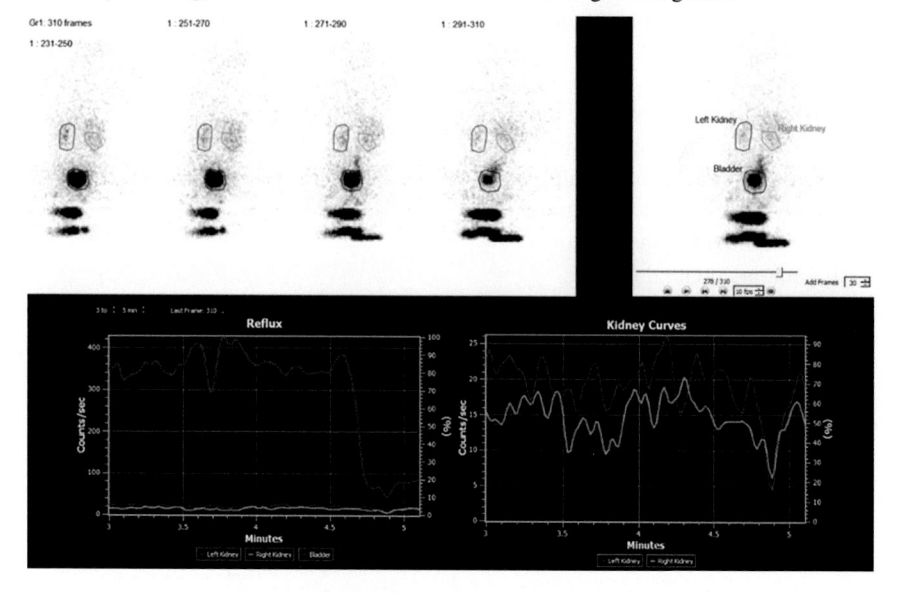

The most appropriate treatment is
A. Cross trigonal reimplantation
B. Hydrodistention Implantation Technique
C. Intermittent catheterisation
D. Loop ureterostomy
E. Vesicostomy

5. A 9-year-old girl presents with recurrent UTI and right flank pain. Her renal ultrasound is normal, and her indirect cystogram showed no reflux. DMSA showed scarring of the right kidney.
The most appropriate next step for management is
A. CT KUB with contrast
B. Cystoscopy
C. Intravenous urogram
D. Magnetic resonance urography
E. Video urodynamics

7.5 Urinary Lithiasis

1. A 2-year-old girl with frequent urinary tract infections, right-sided flank pain and haematuria had an ultrasound scan.

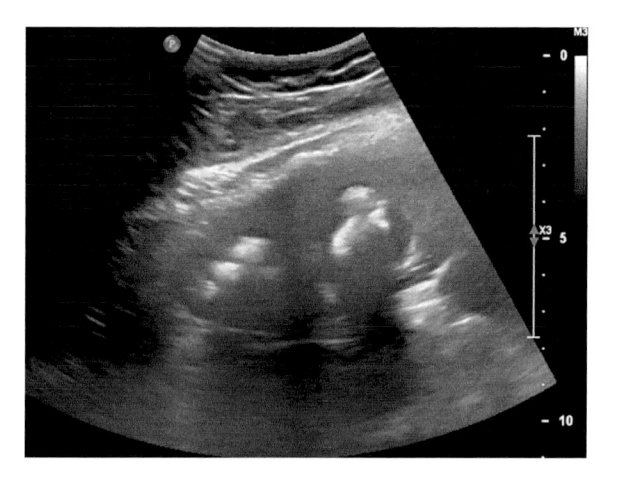

   The pathogenesis is
   A. Dehydration
   B. High urinary pH
   C. Hypercalciuria
   D. Hyperoxaluria
   E. Hyperphosphatemia

2. A 4-year-old boy with Lesch-Nyhan Syndrome presented to the Emergency department with pain in the right flank and haematuria lasting 4 days. He had passed a small stone per urethra. His ultrasound scan is normal.
   Which is the appropriate management
   A. Ammonium chloride
   B. Cysteamine
   C. Hydrochlorothiazide
   D. Lumasiran
   E. Xanthine oxidase inhibitor

3. A 3-year-old child has the most common inheritable cause of kidney stone disease. The medication used to reduce renal stone formation is
   A. Allopurinol
   B. Ammonium chloride
   C. Hydrochlorothiazide
   D. Lumasiran
   E. Tiopronin

4. A 14-year-old girl with no background metabolic history presents with right flank pain and haematuria for a week. There is no family history of renal stones. What is the most sensitive test for diagnosing renal stones?
   A. Abdominal x-ray
   B. Intravenous urogram
   C. Magnetic resonance urogram
   D. Non-contrast helical CT
   E. Ultrasound
5. A 9-year-old girl with cystinuria was found to have a 4 mm renal stone on an ultrasound scan. There is no hydronephrosis. She is asymptomatic.
   Which of the following can be used as medical expulsive therapy?
   A. Ammonium chloride
   B. Hydrochlorothiazide
   C. Potassium Citrate
   D. Tamsulosin
   E. Tiopronin
6. A 14-year-old girl with no background metabolic history presents with right flank pain and haematuria for a week. There is no family history of renal stones. Ultrasound shows a 20 mm stone in the renal pelvis in the lower pole calyx.
   Which is the most appropriate treatment?
   A. Open nephrolithotomy
   B. Percutaneous nephrolithotomy
   C. Retrograde intrarenal surgery
   D. Shockwave lithotripsy
   E. Ureteroscopy
7. A 14-year-old boy with no background metabolic history presents with left flank pain and haematuria for a week. There is no family history of renal stones. A non-contrast CT was performed. The calculus measures 15 mm in diameter.

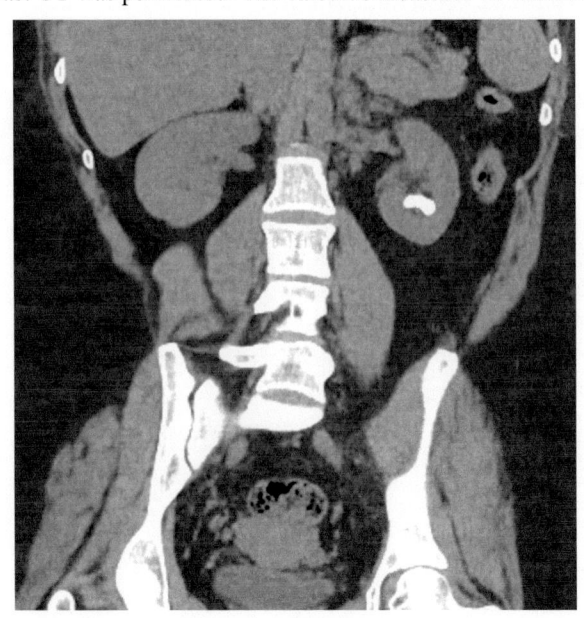

7.6 Renal Infection

Which is the most appropriate treatment according to EAU/ESPU guidelines?
A. Open nephrolithotomy
B. Percutaneous nephrolithotomy
C. Retrograde intrarenal surgery
D. Shockwave lithotripsy
E. Ureteroscopy

8. A 15-year-old girl with spina bifida had bladder neck reconstruction, ileocystoplasty and Mitrofanoff 4 years ago. She developed a 3cm calculus in the bladder. Which is the most appropriate treatment
   A. Endoscopic extraction through Mitrofanoff
   B. Endoscopic extraction through the urethra
   C. Laparoscopic cystolithotomy
   D. Percutaneous cystolithotomy
   E. Shockwave lithotripsy

7.6 Renal Infection

1. A 4-year-old girl presents with first episode of urinary tract infection. Urine grows Proteus mirabilis.
   Which investigation is necessary
   A. DMSA scan 4 to 6 months
   B. MAG3 renogram
   C. MCUG
   D. Ultrasound during the acute infection
   E. Ultrasound within 6 weeks

2. A 15-year-old girl presents with flank and abdominal pain, fever, and weight loss. A CT scan was obtained

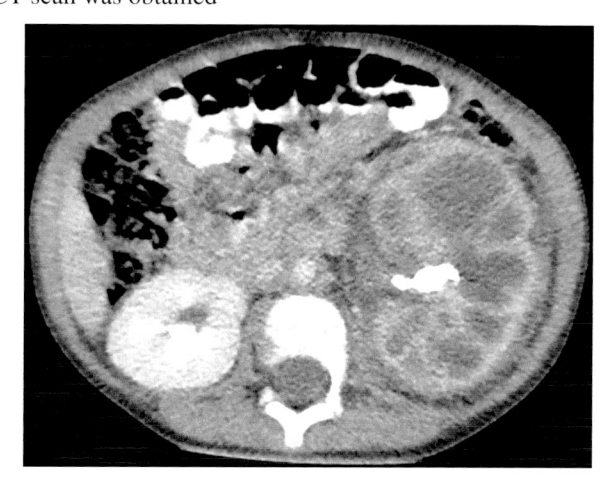

Which is the most appropriate treatment?
A. Nephrectomy
B. Nephrostomy
C. Percutaneous drainage
D. PCNL
E. Ureteric stent

3. A 15-year-old girl presents with right flank pain and pyrexia. Urine dip suggests UTI. CT scan showed a patchy reduction of contrast uptake in the right kidney
Which is the most appropriate initial treatment?
A. Amoxicillin
B. Cefalexin
C. Co-amoxiclav
D. Nitrofurantoin
E. Trimethoprim

4. A 10-year-old diabetic boy presents with right flank pain with turbid burning urination. A CT scan was obtained [Case courtesy of Khairy Abdella, Radiopaedia.org, rID: 39951].

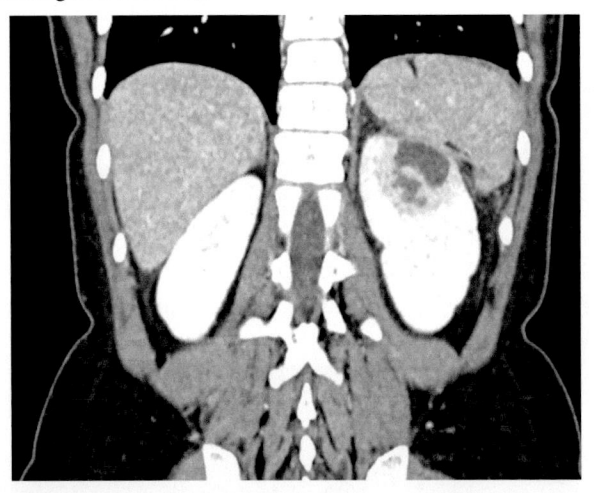

Which is the most appropriate next step in the management?
A. DMSA scan
B. MAG3 renogram
C. Nephrectomy
D. Percutaneous drainage
E. Ureteric stent

7.7 Duplication of Renal Tract

1. A 5-month-old girl is admitted to the hospital with a urinary tract infection with pyrexia. The USS demonstrated a right duplex kidney. The image of the bladder is displayed

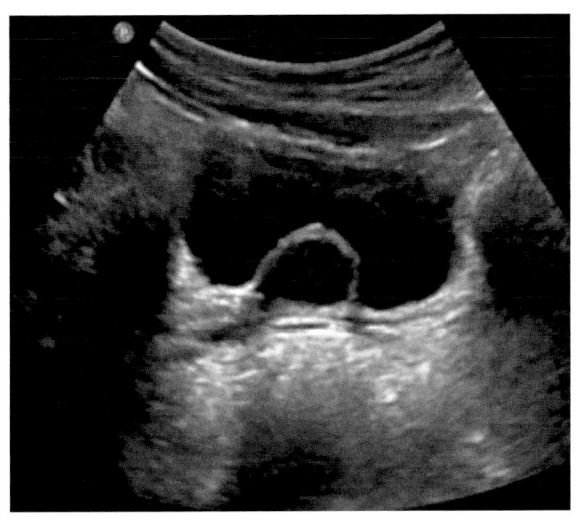

   Which is the most appropriate management
   A. Cystoscopic puncture
   B. Heminephroureterectomy
   C. Ureteric clipping
   D. Ureteric reimplant
   E. Ureterostomy

2. A 7-year-old girl presented with primary urinary incontinence. She can pass urine with a normal urinary stream and has normal perineal and back examinations. Her USS is displayed.

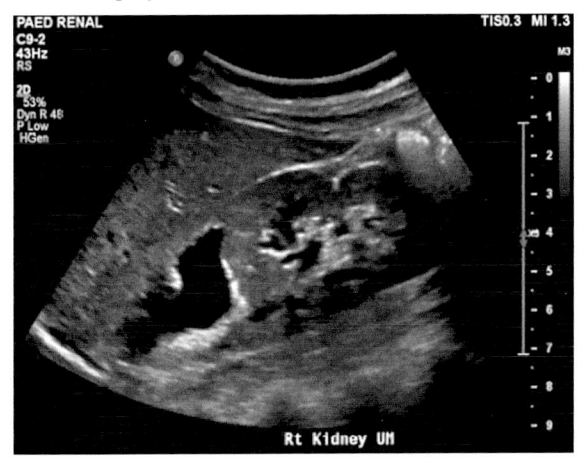

The next step in her management is?
A. Cystoscopy
B. DMSA scan
C. Examination under anaesthetic
D. MCUG
E. MR Urography

3. An 18-month-old girl presents with recurrent UTIs. There was an antenatal left hydronephrosis. MCUG showed reflux in a partial duplex left ureter. Contrast in the collecting system was retained after voiding. DMSA showed 20% function in the left kidney with uniform distribution in the upper and lower poles. Cystoscopy showed single ureteric orifices bilaterally.
   What is the most appropriate management?
   A. Nephrostomy
   B. Heminephrectomy
   C. Ureteric reimplant
   D. Ureteroureterostomy
   E. Vesicostomy

4. A 4-year-old girl presents with UTI. Her ultrasound is displayed.

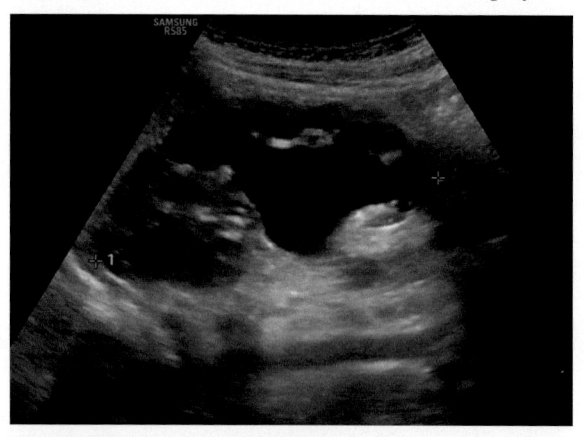

   The most appropriate next step in management is
   A. Heminephrectomy
   B. Injection of Deflux
   C. JJ stent
   D. Pyeloplasty
   E. Reimplantation

5. A 7-day-old girl has a cystic structure extruding from her vagina. She has not passed urine for 18 hours. The USS demonstrates a hydronephrotic upper pole of the right kidney.
   The next step of the management is
   A. CT abdomen
   B. Tumour markers
   C. Urinary catheterisation.
   D. Puncture
   E. Excision

6. A 5-year-old boy has recurrent epididymitis. His ultrasound showed left hydronephrosis, and a DMSA scan showed 20% function on the left. MCUG was performed

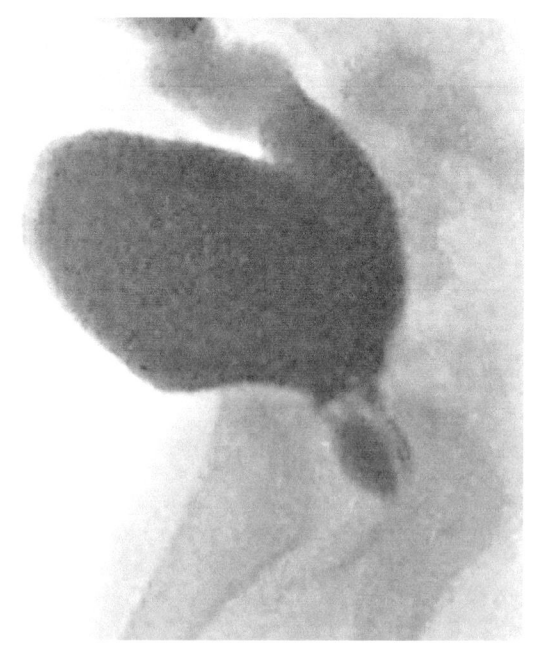

Which is the most appropriate treatment?
A. Injection of Deflux
B. Puncture of ureterocele
C. Ureteric reimplantation
D. Ureteroureterostomy
E. Vasectomy

7.8 Disorders of Bladder Function

1. A 6-year-old girl with urgency, frequency and urge incontinence, has not improved after urotherapy and a bowel programme.
   Which is the most appropriate next step of management?
   A. Anticholinergics
   B. Botulinum Toxin A injections to detrusor
   C. Posterior tibial nerve stimulation
   D. Selective serotonin reuptake inhibitors
   E. Transcutaneous Electrical Nerve Stimulation

2. A 6-year-old girl with recurrent UTI demonstrates interrupted ("staccato") voiding on uroflowmetry.
   Which is the most appropriate treatment
   A. Alpha blocker
   B. Anticholinergics
   C. Biofeedback
   D. Posterior tibial nerve stimulation
   E. Transcutaneous Electrical Nerve Stimulation
3. A 9-year-old girl has recurrent UTIs. She passes urine once or twice a day. She has to strain to complete voiding. Uroflowmetry showed a low flow rate, and video urodynamics showed low voiding pressures and high post-void residual volume.
   Which is the most appropriate treatment
   A. Alpha blocker
   B. Anticholinergics
   C. Clean intermittent catheterisation
   D. Posterior tibial nerve stimulation
   E. Selective serotonin reuptake inhibitors
4. A 15-year-old girl has large volume urinary leakage that only occurs with giggling or laughing but at no other time. Her urodynamic examination is normal. Her symptoms started when she was 9. A trial of anticholinergic medication was ineffective.
   Which is the most appropriate treatment
   A. Desmopressin
   B. Imipramine
   C. Mirabegron
   D. Methylphenidate
   E. Sertraline
5. A 15-year-old girl has involuntary leakage of urine on exertion, sneezing or coughing. 3 months of supervised pelvic floor muscle training was ineffective. Urodynamic study confirms genuine stress incontinence.
   Which is the most appropriate treatment
   A. Altemeier procedure
   B. Burch procedure
   C. Clam procedure
   D. Foley procedure
   E. Kelly procedure
6. A 10-day-old female had closure of open spina bifida at day 2 of life. The indwelling catheter was removed 3 days ago. Ultrasound shows no hydronephrosis.
   Which is the most appropriate immediate management of the bladder
   A. CIC
   B. CIC and Oxybutynin
   C. CIC, Oxybutynin and Prophylactic trimethoprim
   D. Oxybutynin
   E. Prophylactic trimethoprim

7. An 8-year-old boy has nocturnal enuresis. Every night, he passes a large volume of urine in the first few hours of the night. He has no urinary symptoms during the day. His fluid intake is optimised, and he is currently using a combination of alarm, desmopressin and tolterodine, but his wetting continues. He is not constipated, and his renal ultrasound is normal.
   Which is the most appropriate next line of management?
   A. Imipramine
   B. Midodrine
   C. Mirabegron
   D. Methylphenidate
   E. Sertraline

7.9 Megaureter and Prune-Belly Syndrome

1. A baby was born with a lax abdominal wall with wrinkled skin and bilateral undescended testis.
   The most common cause of perinatal death is
   A. Birth asphyxia
   B. Cardiac failure
   C. Pulmonary hypoplasia
   D. Uremia
   E. Sepsis
2. A 2-month-old baby girl had an ultrasound scan after a UTI, which showed a right distal ureter measuring 10 mm and SFU grade 1 hydronephrosis in the right kidney.
   The most appropriate management is
   A. Acute DMSA
   B. Follow-up renal ultrasound
   C. MAG 3 scan
   D. Ureteric reimplantation
   E. Ureteric stent
3. A male newborn has a lax abdominal wall and bilateral impalpable testis. Antenatally, bilateral hydronephrosis was identified.
   Urodynamics, if performed in future, is expected to show
   A. Hyper-compliant bladder with a large capacity
   B. Hyper-compliant bladder with a normal capacity
   C. Noncompliant bladder with a small capacity
   D. Normal compliant bladder with a large capacity
   E. Normal compliant bladder with a normal capacity

4. A 3-month-old baby with Prune Belly Syndrome has bilateral hydroureteronephrosis with good renal function
   The most appropriate next step for management is
   A. CIC
   B. Prophylactic antibiotics
   C. Serial ultrasound scan
   D. Ureteric reimplant
   E. Vesicostomy
5. A child has Eagle-Barrett Syndrome
   The gene associated with this condition is also associated with
   A. Autosomal dominant polycystic kidney
   B. Crossed fused renal ectopia
   C. Duplex kidneys
   D. Horseshoe kidney
   E. Multicystic dysplastic kidney
6. MAG3 renogram was performed on a 3-month-old girl with antenatal hydronephrosis showed Right VUJ obstruction with 27% differential function. The maximum diameter of the ipsilateral distal ureter is 7mm on ultrasound.
   What is the most appropriate next step in management
   A. Conservative
   B. Cutaneous ureterostomy
   C. Endoscopic balloon dilatation
   D. JJ-stenting
   E. Refluxing ureterocystotomy

7.10 Bladder and Cloacal Exstrophy

1. The most consistent ultrasound finding in antenatal scans of bladder exstrophy is
   A. Difficulties determining the sex
   B. Lower abdominal mass
   C. Low-set umbilicus
   D. Non-visualization of the bladder
   E. Separation of the pubic rami
2. The deformity of the pelvis seen on x-ray of children with exstrophy is known as
   A. Fishtail deformity
   B. Lobster claw sign
   C. Manta ray sign
   D. Scallop sign
   E. Shrimp sign

3. A 3-year-old child who had bladder exstrophy repaired as a baby has been suffering from recurrent episodes of epididymoorchitis for the past year.
   The most appropriate treatment is
   A. Ciprofloxacin for 10 days
   B. Doxycycline for 14 days
   C. Prophylactic trimethoprim
   D. Suprapubic catheter
   E. Vasectomy
4. A baby was born with cloacal exstrophy
   The most appropriate initial surgery for the bowel is
   A. Caecostomy
   B. End colostomy
   C. PSARP
   D. Pull through
   E. Split ileostomy
5. A 4-year-old girl has primary urinary incontinence. On examination, a bifid clitoris was found.
   The most appropriate initial surgery is
   A. Bilateral ureterostomy
   B. Reconstruction, augmentation and Mitrofanoff
   C. Single-stage reconstruction
   D. Staged reconstruction
   E. Suprapubic catheter

7.11 Hypospadias

1. A 3-year-old boy has a weak urinary stream and difficulty in urination. He had hypospadias surgery when he was one and a half years old. Uroflometry showed a flat curve.
   The most appropriate initial treatment is
   A. Inlay buccal mucosal graft
   B. Internal urethrotomy
   C. Meatoplasty
   D. Suprapubic catheter
   E. Urethral dilatation
2. A newborn was born with hypospadias and aniridia.
   He is at increased risk of developing
   A. Germ cell tumours
   B. Hepatoblastoma
   C. Leukaemia
   D. Neuroblastoma
   E. Wilms Tumour

3. A 9-year-old child has non-retractile foreskin. He never had balanitis. There is no scarring.
   The most appropriate treatment is
   A. Active retraction
   B. Circumcision
   C. Preputioplasty
   D. Reassurance
   E. Topical steroids
4. A 1-year-old child has a significant ventral chordee with an apical meatus. After degloving and the Nesbit procedure, the chordee persists.
   The next surgical step is
   A. Meatal-based flap
   B. Rotation Dartos flap
   C. Staged urethroplasty
   D. Urethral plate transection
   E. Ventral corporotomy
5. A 1-year-old child presents who had single-stage hypospadias repair 6 months ago developed a fistula.
   The surgical treatment will mainly depend on
   A. Location of fistula
   B. Status of distal urethra
   C. Size of fistula
   D. Type of hypospadias
   E. Type of repair
6. The most common cause of sexual dissatisfaction in adult males who had hypospadias surgery in childhood is
   A. Curvature
   B. Painful erection
   C. Penile size
   D. Reduced sensation
   E. Weak ejaculation

7.12 Disorders of Sexual Development

1. A newborn with genotype 46XY has a 21-hydroxylase deficiency.
   The most common phenotype is
   A. Hyperpigmentation
   B. Hypospadias
   C. Normal
   D. Penile enlargement
   E. Undescended testis

7.12 Disorders of Sexual Development

2. A baby has the most common form of 46XX DSD
   Lifelong replacement of the following is required in all cases
   A. Ethinylestradiol
   B. Fludrocortisone
   C. Hydrocortisone
   D. Somatropin
   E. Testosterone

3. A mother who had a previous baby with severe congenital adrenal hyperplasia confirmed a new pregnancy.
   Maternal dexamethasone to prevent virilisation should be started
   A. After chorionic villus sampling
   B. After fetal blood sampling
   C. After 20-week anomaly scan
   D. At the third trimester
   E. Immediately

4. A 15-year-old girl with typical secondary sexual characteristics presents with primary amenorrhoea. MRI showed an absent uterus.
   The most common associated anomaly is
   A. Cardiac defects
   B. Hearing impairment
   C. Limb anomalies
   D. Renal dysplasia
   E. Vertebral defects

5. A 14-year-old girl is investigated for delayed puberty. Her genotype is 45XY. Bilateral streak gonads were found on Laparoscopy.
   The next step in management is
   A. Bilateral gonadectomy
   B. Genitoplasty
   C. Growth hormone
   D. Oestrogen replacement
   E. Vaginal dilatation

6. During unilateral inguinal herniotomy in an 8-year-old female, you encounter a gonad that appears to be a testis
   The most appropriate management is
   A. Biopsy of the gonad
   B. Explore contralateral gonad
   C. No intervention to gonad
   D. Removal of both gonads
   E. Removal of the gonad

7. A 13-year-old girl presents with delayed puberty and a hand deformity. X-ray of the hand showed a short 4th metacarpal on both sides.
   The most common cause of mortality in later life is
   A. Aortic dissection
   B. Liver failure
   C. Malignancy
   D. Pneumonia
   E. Urosepsis

7.13 Posterior Urethral Valves and Urethral Abnormalities

1. A 3-month-old boy presents with a lower abdominal mass. Ultrasound showed a big bladder with a large residual volume. MCUG was performed [Case courtesy: A Cherian https://pediatricurologybook.com/book/chapters/04-25_duplex-urethral-anomalies-and-syringocoele/]

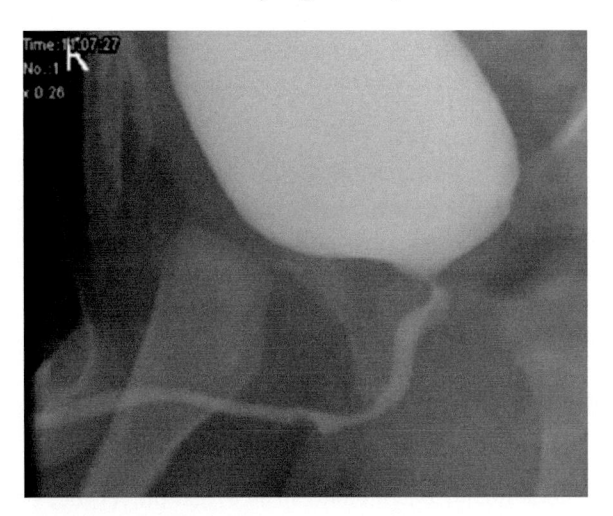

   The most a.ppropriate treatment is
   A. Endoscopic incision
   B. Intermittent catheterisation
   C. Perineal urethrostomy
   D. Urethral dilatation
   E. Vesicostomy

7.13 Posterior Urethral Valves and Urethral Abnormalities

2. In a baby with prune belly syndrome, the shaft of the penis swells up during voiding. The parents have to squeeze out urine from the penis. An MCUG was performed. [Case courtesy: MS Ansari https://pediatricurologybook.com/book/chapters/04-27_prune-belly-syndrome/]

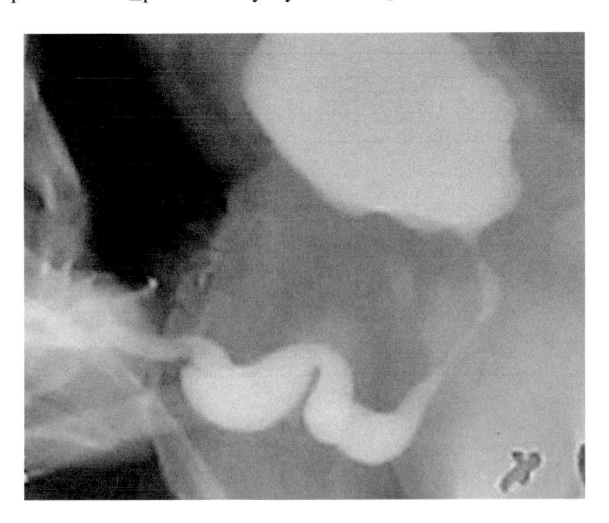

   The most appropriate treatment is
   A. Endoscopic incision
   B. Perineal urethrostomy
   C. Reduction urethroplasty
   D. Urethral dilatation
   E. Vesicostomy

3. Megacystis, oligohydramnios, and potter sequence were seen on an antenatal scan of a male fetus.
   The next step in the management is:
   A. Amnio infusion
   B. Fetal surgery
   C. Steriods
   D. Termination
   E. Vesico amniotic shunt

4. A baby boy is born with urethral atresia after a successful vesicoamniotic shunt. Associated conditions to look for include
   A. Beckwith Wiedeman syndrome
   B. Di George syndrome
   C. Down syndrome
   D. Patau syndrome
   E. Turner's syndrome

5. A male infant with antenatal hydronephrosis was born at 31 weeks of gestation weighing 1.8 Kg. His postnatal ultrasound image of the bladder is displayed. A 5 Fr urinary catheter was passed with difficulty.

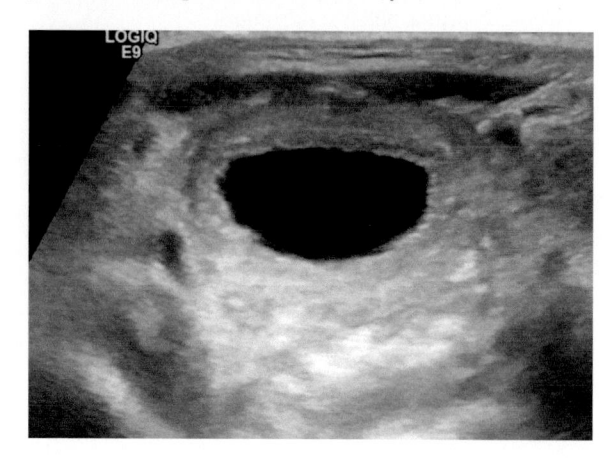

The next step in the management is
   A. Cystoscopic ablation
   B. Ureterostomy
   C. Urethral dilatation
   D. Urethrostomy
   E. Vesicostomy
6. The best prognostic factor in children with posterior urethral valves is
   A. Beta-2 microglobulin on fetal urine analysis
   B. Bilateral high-grade vesicoureteric reflux
   C. Daytime urinary incontinence at 5 yrs of age
   D. Nadir creatinine at 1 yr of age
   E. Oligohydramnios on antenatal scans
7. A 1 yr old baby boy has had ablation of posterior urethral valves on D5 of life. His repeat USS of kidneys shows increasing hydroureteronephrosis.
   The most common aetiology is
   A. Bladder neck hypertrophy
   B. Incomplete ablation of valves
   C. Secondary VUJ obstruction
   D. Urethral stricture post-ablation
   E. Valve bladder syndrome

Answers

Chapter 1 Fetal Medicine

1: C [Most hyperechoic bowel resolves spontaneously]
2: A [Amniocentesis is usually carried out between the 15th and 20th weeks of pregnancy. CVS is usually carried out between the 11th and 14th weeks]
3: B [This is Twin-Twin Transfusion Syndrome. Fetoscopic laser photocoagulation is the treatment]
4: C [FETO performed at 27–30 weeks of gestation]
5: E [Bladder diameter and AFI is normal]
6: C [Steroids and fetal surgery is for microcystic, EXIT is after 32 weeks]
7: A [MOMS trial]
8: C [Reports from UCSF and CHOP Fetal Medicine Unit]

Chapter 2 Paediatric Trauma

1: D [APLS: 10 ml/Kg normal saline bolus; weight = 2 × (age +4)]
2: B [APLS: Child unstable after 40 ml/Kg resuscitation, weight 40 kg Wt = (3 × age) + 7]
3: A [APLS]
4: D [Early distal pancreatectomy for body and tail transections have best outcomes]
5: E [APSA Solid Organ Injury Guidelines 2019]
6: A [APLS: Hypocapnoea and hypercarbia are indications of immediate intubation in head injury]
7: A [NICE guidelines (CG176) Head injury: assessment and early management]
8: B [APLS Front of torso 13%, 1-year-old weight 10 kg, Additional fluid = %xWtx3 modified Parkland formula]
9: C [Mainly adult literature]
10: B [Eastern Association for the Surgery of Trauma guidance]

Chapter 3.1 Wilms' Tumour

1: C [WAGR 11p13]
2: C [Stage III intermediate risk]
3: A [Children with WTI have a high risk of postoperative ESRD. Therefore any normal kidney tissue should be spared. Chemo beyond 12 weeks does not improve outcome]
4: E [Radical dissection does not improve survival, and the tumour is chemo and radiosensitive. Aorta is considered as midline. Therefore, inter-aorto-caval nodes belong to the right side. However, inter-aorto-caval nodes are sampled for both Right and Left-sided tumours]
5: B [See recurrent WT risk groups]
6: B [Umbrella Protocol]
7: C [Clear cell renal cell carcinoma in Von Hippel-Lindau (VHL) disease: Umbrella protocol]
8: A [Malignant rhabdoid tumour of the kidney associated with primary or secondary CNS tumours]

Chapter 3.2 Neuroblastoma

1: C [Opsoclonus-myoclonus-ataxia syndrome (OMAS) with primary abdominal neuroblastoma]
2: A [Tissue diagnosis is necessary]
3: B [CCLG guidance on relapse]
4: D [CCLG: Initial treatment is steroids and emergency chemotherapy. Laminectomy is only for rapidly progressive signs. Emergency chemotherapy should not be delayed for obtaining tissue diagnosis]
5: E [CCLG: Infants diagnosed <3 months old with localised adrenal masses <5cm in diameter, suspicious of neuroblastoma do not necessarily require a biopsy or surgical resection]
6: A [Abdominal compartment syndrome: this is due to hepatomegaly. The primary tumour is usually tiny, and resection is unlikely to help]
7: B [Ascitis is not IDRF. No IDRF: primary resection]
8: A [SIOPEN LINES group 7]

Chapter 3.3 Tumours of the Liver

1: E [Haemangioendothelioma: Radiation therapy is usually avoided because of angiosarcomatous degeneration]
2: B [Mesenchymal hamartoma: risk of undifferentiated embryonal sarcoma if not wholly excised]
3: D [Appears to be Focal nodular hyperplasia. However, because of the oncological history, biopsy to exclude tumour recurrence is essential]

4: B [Hepatoblastoma, APC gene, colonic cancer]
5: C [Beckwith-Wiedemann syndrome: higher adrenal cortical carcinoma but not pheochromocytoma]
6: A [Multifocal lesion not resectable, Low AFP not chemo sensitive]
7: C [Hepatocellular carcinoma in –tyrosinemia]
8: E [If β-catenin activated Hepatocellular Adenoma (β-HCA) is confirmed, resection should be considered regardless of tumour size]

Chapter 3.4 Paediatric Gastrointestinal Tumours

1: D [BSG and ACG guidelines. Chemotherapy based on the histology grade]
2: B [Carney triad: Surgery for pulmonary chondromas is indicated only in case of impaired lung function]
3: E [Burkitt Lymphoma. CCLG Guideline for management of mature B-cell non-Hodgkin lymphoma: CND MRI only if neurological symptoms]
4: B [National Cancer Institute PDQ]
5: E [Juvenile Polyposis Syndrome: ESPGHAN position paper]
6: C [Turcot Syndrome type 2]
7: E [Gardner Syndrome: colectomy if 20–30 polyps seen]
8: C [Familial Adenomatous Polyposis: ESPGHAN position paper]
9: A [Surgery is rarely indicated in Large-cell calcifying Sertoli cell tumours in PJS]

Chapter 3.5 Rhabdomyosarcoma

1: E [In prostatic RMS, LN sampling is only performed if enlarged nodes are detected on imaging]
2: C [European Paediatric Soft Tissue Sarcoma Study Group guidelines]
3: A [Only LN sampling is needed, not formal resection]
4: A [If R0 is achievable, it should be attempted before any other treatment]
5: B [EPSSG: Extremity tumours with unfavourable characteristics (e.g. fusion-positive) will require radiotherapy independent of the surgical margins achieved]

Chapter 3.6 Germ Cell Tumours

1: C [No anal stenosis on MR, the small solid presacral mass would suggest a teratoma which can be excised using a posterior sagittal approach]
2: A [Biopsy, Chemotherapy and surgery for delayed diagnosis of SCT]
3: D [AFP is elevated in malignant recurrences, and CA 125 is elevated in mature or immature recurrences. CEA is usually not helpful for SCT recurrences]

4: E [86% Mediastinal teratomas are benign, so screening for brain metastasis is not routinely performed. Primary surgery or delayed surgery after biopsy and chemotherapy are legitimate options for this size tumour. Screening for Klinefelter syndrome is necessary]
5: A [Fetiform teratoma]
6: A [Growing teratoma syndrome]

Chapter 3.7 Ovarian Tumours

1: A [BritSPAG guidance: conservative till 7 cm]
2: E [BritSPAG guidance]
3: B [BritSPAG guidance]
4: D [Contralateral ovarian biopsy is only recommended if there are suspicious areas]
5: A [The cyst would spontaneously resolve when the child is euthyroid]
6: D
7: B [Juvenile granulosa cell tumor]
8: E [Ovarian sparing surgery for benign ovarian fibroma in nevoid basal cell carcinoma syndrome]
9: A [Sertoli-Leydig cell tumours or steroid cell tumours]
10: A [Gliomatosis peritonei is benign, and biopsy is needed to confirm diagnosis]
11: B [Testis produces hormones that help girls with CAIS develop a normal female body shape without hormone treatment]

Chapter 3.8 Testicular Tumours

1: B [Testicular epidermoid cyst]
2: B [Radiotherapy not in CCLG protocol for germ cell tumours]
3: C [Leydig Cell Tumors: Normal Histology]
4: A [CCLG]
5: A [EAU guidance]

Chapter 3.9 Adrenal Tumours

1: E [Start alpha-blocker to control symptoms. Biopsy not indicated in pheochromocytoma]
2: D [In MEN 2A, pheochromocytoma can be bilateral and multicentric but of adrenal in origin]
3: A [VHL-related pheochromocytoma usually does not produce adrenaline or its metabolite, metanephrine]
4: B [Nodular adrenal hyperplasia: bilateral adrenalectomy and permanent postoperative mineralocorticoid and glucocorticoid replacement]

Answers

5: B [Lung Carcinoid]
6: C [Adrenal insufficiency resulting from bilateral adrenalectomy is more challenging to manage than hyperaldosteronism]
7: A [Adrenal haemorrhage]
8: D [Adrenal carcinoma is not radiosensitive]

Chapter 3.10 Tumours of the Lung and Chest Wall

1: D [Primary disease has to be treated first]
2: A [Complete excision prevents recurrence]
3: D [Carney Triad]
4: C [Carcinoid with ectopic ACTH]
5: B [Usually surgery, but this solid mass is too large for primary excision]
6: C [Most pulmonary metastasis would resolve with chemotherapy]

Chapter 4.1 Craniofacial Anomalies

1: D [The woman has Apert Syndrome, which is autosomal dominant]
2: C [To avoid intracranial hypertension, which has been linked to brain damage, optic nerve compression, and cognitive impairment]
3: B [To prevent elevation of intracranial pressure and its attendant consequences, improve re-ossification of calvarial bone defects, and prevent the need for a more extensive surgical correction]
4: D
5: D

Chapter 4.2 Salivary Glands

1: C [It has a minimal recurrence]
2: A [Parotid infantile hemangioma usually resolves spontaneously]
3: E [MRI is the best soft tissue detail of the salivary glands, and it is the only imaging technique that can delineate the facial nerve anatomy within the parotid glands]
4: B [Phleomorphic adenoma]

Chapter 4.3 Lymph Node Disorders

1: D [Kawasaki disease]
2: B [Any supraclavicular lymph node enlargement is a worrying sign]
3: B [Excision is the treatment of choice for atypical mycobacterial infection of the lymph node]
4: E [To rule out mediastinal lymphadenopathy]

Chapter 4.4 Childhood Diseases of the Thyroid and Parathyroid Glands

1: B [Can be malignancy]
2: C
3: E [Can also be in the forearm]
4: D [All 4 parathyroid glands are affected]
5: A [100% will develop medullary carcinoma of thyroid if not removed]
6: C [American Thyroid Association Guidelines: recommendation 9]

Chapter 4.5 Neck Cysts and Sinuses

1: D [They enlarge very rapidly, and a C section is recommended]
2: A [Surgery is usually the treatment of choice but ethanol ablation is the choice for these high-risk patients]
3: B [Thymic cyst]
4: D
5: A [Early surgical excision is the treatment of choice for midline cervical cleft]

Chapter 5.1 Disorders of the Breast

1: D
2: A
3: B [Klinefelter's syndrome]
4: A [Secretory carcinoma: Cure rate is excellent with surgical excision even for local recurrence]
5: C [Juvenile papillomatosis is benign]
6: B [Breast lumps in Beckwith is usually benign fibroadenoma. Excision needed as rapidly growing]
7: C
8: C [Hereditary Breast and Ovarian Cancer Syndrome (HBOC)]
9: A [Benign premature thelarche]
10: B [S.aureus: penicillin]

Chapter 5.2 Congenital Chest Wall Deformities

1: B [The patient has cerebro costo mandibular syndrome]
2: D [Jarcho Levin syndrome is an autosomal recessive disorder]
3: A [Jeuene syndrome]
4: C

Answers

5: C [Poland syndrome]
6: C
7: D
8: C

Chapter 5.3 Congenital Diaphragmatic Hernia and Eventration

1: D
2: A
3: D
4: C [Gastric fixation anomalies are common in eventration and may present with gastric volvulus]
5: C [Morgagni hernia: Leaving the sac alone does not have long-term consequences]
6: C [Total study: Severe CDH. FETO best for survival to discharge]
7: C [Pulmonary hypertension]

Chapter 5.4 Congenital Lung Malformations

1: A [CPAM volume ratio is 0.11 and can safely be observed]
2: C
3: D [The lesion is classic of CPAM, and regular follow-up with ultrasound is indicated]
4: E [Hydrops]
5: C [Nitric Oxide induction increases mediastinal shift in the lung owing to its rapid spread in the closed cavity]
6: A [CLE: Massive distention of alveolar spaces, but no tissue destruction]
7: A
8: B
9: A

Chapter 5.5 Oesophageal Rupture and Perforation

1: A
2: B
3: B [Oesophageal perforation]
4: E [Pneumomediastinum: oesophageal perforation]
5: B [Leaking for 6 weeks]
6: D [Aorto-oesophageal fistula]
7: E

Chapter 5.6 Oesophageal Atresia

1: E
2: C [Aortic arch is more consistent with the alignment of the liver]
3: D [CHARGE]
4: A
5: C
6: D
7: B [Oesophageal replacement needed once oesophagostomy performed]
8: A [A Boix-Ochoa score of less than 11.99 is considered normal. So symptoms are due to tracheomalacia and not reflux]
9: B
10: D

Chapter 5.7 Foreign Body Ingestion

1: C
2: A
3: A [Aorto-oesophageal fistula]
4: A
5: D
6: A [To exclude strictures]
7: B
8: B

Chapter 5.8 Gastroesophageal Reflux Disease

1: B [Hypomagnesemia is a severe side effect of prolonged use of PPI]
2: C [Severe interaction: Omeprazole slightly to moderately increases the exposure to Citalopram. Manufacturer advises monitor and adjust dose.]
3: B [Pediatric Gastroesophageal Reflux Clinical Practice Guidelines: Joint Recommendations of the North American Society for Pediatric Gastroenterology, Hepatology, and Nutrition and the European Society for Pediatric Gastroenterology, Hepatology, and Nutrition]
4: A [Eosinopilic oesophagitis]
5: E [BSG guidelines <3 cm]
6: C [All others anterior wrap]
7: D [Carobel]

Chapter 6.1 Congenital Defects of the Abdominal Wall

1: A [A. Hypomethylation most common as well as maternal inheritance]
2: B [Artificial insemination is required]
3: B
4: C
5: D [gastroschisis prone to premature labour. Planned institutional delivery is needed in tertiary centres.]
6: C [Component separation]

Chapter 6.2 Inguinal Hernias and Hydroceles

1: C [Same as the cremasteric reflex]
2: B [Ilioinguinal nerve motor supply: internal oblique and transversus abdominis]
3: B [Cremasteric artery is a branch of the inferior epigastric artery]
4: A [most will not develop a symptomatic hernia
5: C [CFTR 7q31. 2]
6: D [Direct hernia after open appendicectomy: Lichtenstein tension-free mesh repair]

Chapter 6.3 Undescended Testis

1: C [NICE CKS]
2: C [NICE CKS]
3: A
4: A
5: E [Reselient looping vas cannot be easily dissected out of the canal – sharp dissection and diathermy are dangerous. Mobilising testis without freeing the vas is not safe either]
6: C [Hydatid of Morgagni attached to the upper pole of the testis is Mullerian remnant, but appendix attached to epididymis is Wolffian duct remnant]
7: C [There is a minimal nonsignificant increase in scrotal temperature on the hydrocele side]
8: C [Testis to be preserved in Klinefelter due to hypogonadism. Shehata cannot be performed in 15yo]

Chapter 6.4 Hypertrophic Pyloric Stenosis

1: D [Redundant pyloric mucosa protruding into the stomach]
2: C [Normal measurements in 3 months]
3: D[Atropine]
4: A[Pyloric atresia]

Chapter 6.5 Bariatric Surgery in Adolescents

1: C [BMI 35 with major comorbidity or BMI 40 with minor comorbidity. NAS 4 or more is a major comorbidity.]
2: B [VSG is the most common procedure]
3: C [34F bougie, short gastric divided, less staple line complications with reinforcement, triangular area of stomach left behind at GO junction]
4: B [Thiamine and Magnessium]

Chapter 6.6 Intestinal Atresia

1: C [Duodenal web: if proximal enterotomy is distal to the web, a tube pushed proximally will not reach the stomach]
2: C[Maternal causes are more common for polyhydramnios]
3: A
4: B
5: C
6: A
7: E [SMA is absent after MCA]

Chapter 6.7 Meconium Ileus

1: B [CFTR ion channel is responsible for apical membrane secretion of chloride and bicarbonate, which is decreased in CF. This in turn, decreases transcellular passive secretion of sodium and water. In contrast, in sweat gland reabsorptive duct epithelium, the channels absorb chloride, causing high sweat chloride in CF.]
2: C [98% male with CV infertile due to congenital bilateral absence of the vas deferens (CBAVD)]
3: A [70% born with no abnormalities]
4: A [Hyperosmolar draws water]
5: E [Fibrosing colonopathy]
6: D [Meconium peritonitis]
7: A
8: B [Rectal biopsy and CF screening must be performed in small left colon]

Answers

Chapter 6.8 Intussusception

1: A
2: C [Malnourished children are considered to have a lower risk of intussusception because of less prominent intestinal lymphoid tissue]
3: E [RotaShield was withdrawn from the market in 1999 for high intussusception rates]
4: A [Peutz-Jeghers Syndrome]
5: C [Incident of intussusception around the jejunal tube is lower if the tip is close to GJ]
6: C

Chapter 6.9 Malrotation

1: C [Malrotation with volvulus in a healthy 4-day-old]
2: D [inverted SMA/SMV relationship is seen in 11% without malrotation, a normal relationship seen in 29% in malrotation]
3: D
4: A [incising the lateral peritoneal reflection of the right colon]
5: D
6: A
7: C

Chapter 6.10 Short Bowel Syndrome

1: C [Increased unabsorbed fatty acids and bile salts bind calcium, resulting in increased oxalate absorption]
2: A [Vancomycin]
3: A [All gastric inhibitory small bowel hormones are decreased]
4: E [Enterohepatic circulation]
5: B [reflux of colonic organism]

Chapter 6.11 Gastrointestinal Bleeding

1: B [Octreotide]
2: C [BSPGHAN]
3: D
4: B [Only acid suppressor]
5: D [Paediatric patients with SMAD4 mutation should be evaluated for hereditary haemorrhagic telangiectasia, including screening and preventative treatment for cerebral and pulmonary AVMs.]
6: E
7: B [Continue breastfeeding]

Chapter 6.12 Alimentary Tract Duplications

1: C
2: D
3: A
4: B
5: D

Chapter 6.13 Polypoid Diseases of the Gastrointestinal Tract

1: D
2: B
3: B
4: C
5: A
6: D
7: D
8: A

Chapter 6.14 Necrotising Enterocolitis

1: A [failure of medical management]
2: C [Damage control]
3: A [Maternal glucocorticoids, indomethacin and magnesium sulphate have been linked]
4: A [Early breastfeeding is protective]
5: A [Klebsiella spp. (Klebsiella pneumoniae, Klebsiella oxytoca), Shigella dysenteriae, Escherichia coli, and Citrobacter koseri were identified as the dominating taxa present in the gut of NEC infants]
6: B
7: C [Lactobacillus and Bifidubacterium are probiotic]
8: B [Multiple strictures]

Chapter 6.15 Inflammatory Bowel Disease

1: E [Oral Vancomycin for *C difficile*]
2: C [NOD2/CARD15: increased severity of ileal disease requiring surgical intervention/reoperation]
3: E [Calprotectin]
4: B [Due to decreased fat absorption]
5: D [Fistula]
6: C [Ileal stricture]

Answers

7: D [Modulen IBD TGF- β]
8: A [Mild disease: Mesalazine for mild and moderate disease]
9: D [Abscess]
10: D

Chapter 6.16 Appendicitis

1: E [PMID: 33896004 DOI: 10.1111/aogs.14165]
2: B [Threadworm]
3: C [9.6 mm appendix tip]
4: C [Accessory appendicular artery]
5: E[Appendectomy alone is sufficient treatment for pediatric appendiceal neuroendocrine tumours regardless of size, position, histology, or nodal or mesenteric involvement, and that right hemicolectomy is unnecessary in children. Routine follow-up imaging and biologic studies were not beneficial (https://www.cancer.gov/types/gi-neuroendocrine-tumors/hp/pediatric-gi-neuroendocrine-treatment-pdq)]

Chapter 6.17 Hirschsprung Disease

1: D[Congenital Central Hypoventilation Syndrome: Haddad syndrome]
2: C [Waardenburg Type 4]
3: C [Rectosigmoid ratio >1: Small left colon. Repeat the enema]
4: D [Absent RAIR is pathognomic of HD]
5: A
6: C [Question mark colon in total colonic HD: initial ileostomy]

Chapter 6.18 Anorectal Malformations

1: D
2: C
3: A [Primary PSARP for air below coccyx <1 cm from the skin]
4: A [Perineal approach enough for rectum below coccyx]
5: A [Perineal fistula]
6: D
7: E [Palpable mass is hydrometrocolpos]
8: C [Pena never observed continence if SI is <0.3]
9: B [83% in perianal fistula: Pena]
10: B
11: A
12: A

Chapter 6.19 Biliary Atresia and Choledochal Cyst

1: E
2: D [Better prognosis in cystic BA; visible ductal structures in the porta does not alter prognosis]
3: B [BASM]
4: B [Biliary atresia]
5: B [Gancyclovir used in CMV infection is a polymerase inhibitor which blocks genome replication]
6: B [No need for cholangiogram if no bile in GB: proceed to Kasai]
7: B [Due to bile reflux. Hepaticojejunostomy preferred for Type 1 choledochal cyst; other options not treatment of choledochal cysts]
8: E [MRI shows Caroli disease. ARPKD and stage 4 CKD will require a renal transplant. Immunosuppression from renal transplant will make cholangitis worse. The only definitive treatment for Caroli disease is a liver transplant]

Chapter 6.20 Gallbladder Disease

1: C
2: B [GB hydrops common in Kawasaki Disease]
3: D [Cholecystectomy for biliary dyskinesia]
4: A [Society of Radiologists in Ultrasound Consensus Conference Recommendations]
5: E [Lower cystic duct insertions have lower CBD stones]
6: E [Low-lying cystic artery, which does not pass through Calot's triangle]
7: A [Not for immediate transplant for 1-year-old with no cirrhosis]
8: A [British Society of Gastroenterology 2016 guideline]
9: C [2020 WSES guidelines. CBD is not dilated in this case for bowel anastomosis]
10: A [Inflammation causing cystic duct obstruction]

Chapter 6.21 Portal Hypertension

1: D [Risk factors for portal vein thrombosis related to UVC: Tip in the portal vein (Liver), blood transfusion, stays longer than a week. T8 in the neonate is IVC and the correct tip position. The tip in RA is not right but is not a risk for PVT. PN is not a proven risk either]
2: D [Budd-Chiari syndrome: B and C are total portal diversions which are not done in any situation]
3: A [Endoscopic treatment of varices necessary even if the bleeding stopped as it is likely to bleed again]
4: B [Liver Transplantation is the only cure for hepatopulmonary syndrome]
5: C [Shunt improves hypersplenism without the risks of splenectomy and will also improve portal hypertension]

Answers

6: D [In the congenital absence of portal vein occlusion, portosystemic shunts would not work]
7: B [ERCP with stenting recommended for dominant CBD stricture of <1.5mm in sclerosing cholangitis]
8: C [BSPGHAN guidance: 7yo is <30 kg so 14Fr, 16Fr for >30 kg]
9: D [BSPGHAN: This is grade 2; multiple grade 2 varices will require banding; treated varices are scoped again in 1–3months]
10: C [Histoacryl glue injection sclerotherapy is the first-line treatment of gastric varices]

Chapter 6.22 The Pancreas

1: B [The annular pancreas is usually (85%) located above the papilla of Vater, 60% asymptomatic, Pancreatitis 16% (adults)]
2: D [Shwachman-Diamond syndrome: Creon (Pancrelipase) for exogenous pancreas insufficiency]
3: D [Fusiform choledochal malformation and non-stenotic long common channel. Treated as choledochal malformation]
4: B [Pancreaticijejunostomy]
5: A [The genetic mutation would dictate the need for imaging. A mutation suggestive of focal or no identified mutation results in need for a PET CT. Mutation consistent with the diffuse disease means no PET CT]
6: A [Biopsy of the tip of the tail to ensure it is not diffuse disease]
7: C [Allow cyst wall to mature before cystgastrostomy]
8: E [VIPoma: Complete surgical resection is the treatment of choice for primary tumours and is usually a distal pancreatectomy]
9: B [Insulinoma: Diaxoxide causes weight gain by fluid retention. Thiazide diuretics are used to treat fluid retention]
10: E [Valproate increases GABA levels]

Chapter 6.23 The Spleen

1: B [Though splenosis is most likely based on the history of trauma, a biopsy is still needed to ensure these are not metastatic deposits. Incidental asymptomatic splenosis does not require any treatment]
2: B [Splenopexy for wandering spleen]
3: D [Fontan circulation is needed in most Right atrial isomerism. Norwood is the first stage]
4: E [Associated anomalies in continuous splenogonadal fusion]
5: E [Pentamidine has no role against echinococcus and is not in WHO treatment for hydatid disease]
6: A [Green book: PCV13 is for under 2years of age]
7: E [British Committee for Standards in Haematology 1996]

8: B [Most children will end up with auto-splenectomy. Prophylactic surgery is only considered in recurrent disease]
9: D [BSH guidance]
10: A [ASH clinical practice guidelines]

Chapter 7.1 Renal Agenesis, Dysplasia, and Cystic Disease

1: B [Ureteric Bud]
2: C [Contralateral VUR]
3: D
4: B [ARPKD: Pulmonary hypoplasia]
5: E [ACE inhibitor – reno-protective]
6: B
7: A
8: B [Microcysts appear hyperechoic due to the cyst walls]
9: D [Congenital hepatic fibrosis (CHF)]

Chapter 7.2 Renal Fusions and Ectopia

1: A [Crossed fused ectopia]
2: A [Horseshoe kidney and Turner syndrome]
3: C [Horseshoe kidney: PCNL preferred, ESWL not reliable in the pelvis, ureteric anatomy variable]
4: A [in 60% cases, there is a separate artery from aorta]

Chapter 7.3 Pelviureteric Junction Obstruction

1: C
2: A
3: D [Most will spontaneously resolve]
4: E [fibrosis with high collagen]
5: C [Already 2 weeks so that stent can be safely removed]
6: E [Nearly 100% renal excretion]
7: C [Dilated non-obstructed system]

Chapter 7.4 Vesicoureteral Reflux

1: A
2: E
3: A [Deflux injection is not usually successful in grade 5 VUR with standing column]

Answers

4: B [Deflux]
5: B [Most likely diagnosis is reflux. The next step is cystoscopic hydrodistension or PIC cystogram]

Chapter 7.5 Urinary Lithiasis

1: B [Huge acoustic shadow suggests staghorn calculus. Urease-producing organisms make the urine alkalotic]
2: E [Allopurinol for urate stones]
3: E [Cystinuria]
4: D [CT most sensitive, but US first line investigation]
5: D [medical expulsive therapy (MET) uses α-blockers (tamsulosin and doxazosin). Tiopronin and Potassium Citrate are preventive]
6: B [PCNL better than ESWL in lower-pole calyx stone – EAU/ESPU guidelines]
7: D [EAU/ESPU guidelines]
8: D [Percutaneous or Open surgery]

Chapter 7.6 Renal Infection

1: A [NICE NG224]
2: A [Xanthogranulomatous pyelonephritis]
3: B [Pyelonephritis NICE]
4: D [Renal abscess]

Chapter 7.7 Duplication of Renal Tract

1: A [Ureteroele]
2: B [To check differential function]
3: C
4: B [Most recent studies suggest Deflux can be effective in duplex]
5: D [Prolapsed ureterocele]
6: C [Single moiety ectopic ureter with reasonable renal function]

Chapter 7.8 Disorders of Bladder Function

1: A [Overactive Bladder]
2: C [Dysfunctional voiding: external sphincter dyssynergia more common]
3: C [Underactive bladder: severe symptoms]
4: D [Giggle incontinence is generally believed to be a neurological (rather than urological) phenomenon]
5: B [Burch colposuspension]

6: B [Neuropathic bladder: Early CIC and oxybutynin are protective. Antibiotics not routinely needed as no hydronephrosis]
7: A [Tricyclics - NICE CG111: Bedwetting in under 19s]

Chapter 7.9 Megaureter and Prune-Belly Syndrome

1: C [Pulmonary hypoplasia as a result of oligohydramnios from reduced fetal urine production from renal dysplasia and urinary tract abnormalities leading to Potter sequence]
2: B
3: A [Prune belly syndrome bladder]
4: B [Prevention of infection is more important than dealing with obstruction for renal preservation]
5: A [CHRM3 gene: Polycystic kidney disease 1]
6: D [VUJ obstruction <40% function needs treatment]

Chapter 7.10 Bladder and Cloacal Exstrophy

1: D
2: C [Diastatic pubic rami in exstrophy]
3: E [Cause of recurrent epididymitis is anatomical]
4: B [Tubularisation of caecum with end colostomy]
5: C [Female epispadias can be corrected in one stage. Augmentation may be needed is some children later in life]

Chapter 7.11 Hypospadias

1: E
2: E [WAGR]
3: D [Physiological phimosis – wait till puberty before any treatment (BMJ best practice)]
4: D [This is usually a form of hypospadias with flimsy distal urethra. Should be treated as hypospadias back to healthy spongiosum-supported urethra]
5: B [Distal urethral stricture, if present, has to be managed first]
6: C

Chapter 7.12 Disorders of Sexual Development

1: C [Most males have no signs of CAH at birth]
2: C [Glucocorticoid in CAH]

Answers

3: E [The virilisation occurs within the first 12 weeks of gestation. The virilisation will have already occurred if one waits to confirm the diagnosis. In this strategy, 7/8 babies will be treated unnecessarily]
4: D [Mayer-Rokitansky-Kuster-Hauser syndrome type II]
5: A [Swyer syndrome: 46, XY complete gonadal dysgenesis. The vagina, uterus, tubes and external genitals are normal. Gonadectomy is performed before HRT due to the risk of cancer]
6: A [CAIS: Biopsy to confirm Testis. Bilateral gonadectomy in performed after puberty]
7: A [Short 4th Metacarpal is found in Turner Syndrome. Aortic aneurysm is common in Turner]

Chapter 7.13 Posterior Urethral Valves and Urethral Abnormalities

1: A [Unruptured syringocele: Urethroscopic laying open]
2: C [Scaphoid megalourethra: urethroplasty similar to hypospadias]
3: E
4: B
5: E [Thick bladder of PUV. At least a size 8 catheter and 2.5 kg weight are needed for cystoscopic ablation. Definitive bladder drainage is recommended while waiting]
6: D
7: E [Bladder function remains problematic even after successful ablation]

GPSR Compliance

The European Union's (EU) General Product Safety Regulation (GPSR) is a set of rules that requires consumer products to be safe and our obligations to ensure this.

If you have any concerns about our products, you can contact us on ProductSafety@springernature.com

In case Publisher is established outside the EU, the EU authorized representative is:

Springer Nature Customer Service Center GmbH
Europaplatz 3
69115 Heidelberg, Germany

Batch number: 08730799

Printed by Printforce, the Netherlands